ᒧ

Is it me or my hormones?

Is it me or my hormones?

Understanding midlife change

Second edition

Dr Margaret Smith & Patricia Michalka

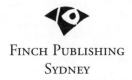

FINCH PUBLISHING
SYDNEY

Is It Me or My Hormones? Understanding midlife change (Second edition)
This edition first published in 2006 in Australia and New Zealand by Finch Publishing Pty
Limited, PO Box 120, Lane Cove, NSW 1595, Australia. ABN 49 057 285 248. This is a
revised edition of *Is It Me or My Hormones? Women in transition*, originally published by Caring
for Women Publications in 2003.

09 08 07 06   8 7 6 5 4 3

National Library of Australia Cataloguing-in-Publication entry

Smith, Margaret.
   Is it me or my hormones? : understanding midlife change.

   2nd ed.
   Bibliography.
   Includes index.
   ISBN 1 876451 74 2.

   1. Menopause - Popular works. 2. Menopause - Hormone
   therapy - Popular works. I. Michalka, Patricia. II. Title.

   618.175

Edited by Kathryn Lamberton
Editorial assistance from Rosemary Peers
Text designed and typeset in Adobe Garamond by J&M Typesetting
Illustrations © 2006 Cathy Wilcox
Cover design by Steve Miller – 154 Design
Cover photography courtesy of Getty Images
Printed by BPA Print Group

Notes: The medical chapters have been written by Dr Margaret Smith. Patricia Michalka has
contributed Chapters 20 and 23 and all the chapters in Part 5 on emotional wellbeing. Margaret
has also drawn on Patricia's expertise in Chapters 2–5 and Chapter 22.

The 'Authors' notes' section at the back of this book contains useful additional information
and references to quoted material in the text. Each reference is linked to the text by its relevant
page number and an identifying line entry.

Disclaimers While every care has been taken in researching and compiling the information in
this book, it is in no way intended to replace other medical advice and counselling. Readers are
encouraged to seek such help as they deem necessary. The authors and publisher specifically
disclaim any liability arising from the application of information in this book.

Every effort has been made by the authors and the publisher to acknowledge copyright material
accurately. However, if any acknowledgement has been inadvertently overlooked, due credit
will be made at the first opportunity.

Other Finch titles can be viewed at **www.finch.com.au**

'Many talk about "holistic" approaches in medicine – but few manage to do it. Here is a book on menopause that truly examines the mind, body and spirit. Menopause is a time of life where not only physical symptoms like hot flushes or aches and pains may need to be addressed, but often hidden issues surface. These may relate to childbearing, fear of death and loss, worries about one's spouse or children and even purpose in life. I particularly enjoyed the chapter on forgiveness. Margaret and Patricia are to be congratulated for producing such a helpful book.'

Dr John Eden, Associate Professor of Reproductive Endocrinology, University of NSW; Director of the Sydney Menopause Centre and the Natural Therapies Unit, Royal Hospital for Women, Sydney

'Much is made in contemporary discussion of the over-medicalisation of the menopause. Margaret Smith and Patricia Michalka are to be commended for a book which is balanced and puts the medical aspects of menopause into overall perspective … I am delighted to see the insistence on individual assessment and holistic management of a woman's problems and a comprehensive coverage of the many changes which can occur at mid-life. The chapter summaries are very helpful.'

Professor Henry Burger AO, FAA, Consultant Endocrinologist, Jean Hailes Foundation for Women's Health, Melbourne, and co-founder of the first menopause clinic at Prince Henry Hospital in 1971

'*Is It Me or My Hormones?* is a veritable street directory of the midlife maze. If you're a menopausal woman, or thinking of becoming one, don't leave home without it.'

Susan Maushart, author of What Women Want Next, Wifework *and* The Mask of Motherhood

Contents

She had not started the menopause, but it would have been no use saying so; it had been useful, apparently, for the family's mythology to have a mother in the menopause. Sometimes she felt like a wounded bird being pecked to death by the healthy birds, or like an animal teased by cruel children.

Doris Lessing, *The Summer before the Dark*

Wholly unprepared, we embark on the second half of life. Thoroughly unprepared, with the false supposition that our truths and ideals will survive as hitherto. But we cannot live the afternoon of life according to the program of life's morning.

Carl Jung (1875–1961)

I look forward to being older, when what you look like becomes less and less an issue and what you are is the point.

Susan Sarandon

Introduction

Over the last seven years or so, the question 'Is HRT dangerous?' has evoked major debate. Media headlines about a possible increase in breast cancer and cardiovascular risk in women on hormone replacement therapy (HRT) have alarmed and confused menopausal women. Many have stopped HRT but are still seeking help for the significant changes that occur around this time. For some women there is a need for appropriate HRT and in taking HRT they need reassurance that improved quality of life need not be at the expense of quantity of life. This book imparts information that should provide this reassurance, including the most up-to-date research on breast cancer and cardiovascular risk.

In the sixties, women in the USA were persuaded to undertake estrogen replacement therapy (ERT) under the catchcry 'feminine forever'. In the seventies, the concern that estrogen alone may increase the risk of cancer of the uterine lining (endometrial cancer) caused doctors to think again about the risk–benefit ratio of hormone therapy. In the eighties, progestogens were introduced and ERT became HRT, meaning that both hormones were given to women during menopause. At that time it was believed that such therapy had positive effects on the cardiovascular system and so would provide primary protection against heart attack and stroke. Studies had already shown that HRT could protect bones from the loss of calcium caused by estrogen deficiency and thus prevent osteoporosis, so many women decided to take HRT long term for all these benefits. It was also believed that HRT could improve brain function.

In the nineties came warnings of a possible increased risk of breast cancer for women on HRT for longer than five years and then studies that showed that HRT given to women who had already had a heart attack or stroke did not give protection against a further stroke. Further studies of older women (who did not have menopausal symptoms) showed that quality of life was not improved for these women by giving HRT and nor did HRT protect against loss of brain function.

All these studies were done on women using the standard HRT therapy in the USA – Premarin and Provera. However, in Australia, lower dose estrogens and different progestogens were prescribed by many doctors.

Today, it is generally believed to be appropriate for women to use HRT short term (i.e. for two to five years) for the relief of classic meno-pause symptoms, but the catchcry 'feminine forever' needs revision. It is important to use HRT judiciously and appropriately, and its use must be based on individual need and assessment.

'Is it *me* or my hormones?' is the question most commonly asked by women in their middle years. One woman in midlife said it all when she exclaimed, 'If it's not menopause then I must be going insane.'

In this book we explain how symptoms due to hormone deficiency need to be differentiated from symptoms with medical or emotional causes so that appropriate treatment can be given.

Hormones begin to change and then decline from 35 to 55 during what is called perimenopause. We have therefore included stories from women of all these ages, not just from women who are going through menopause.

In the medical world, before 1960, menopause was hardly mentioned. Now it is acknowledged, although some critics believe that the medical profession has attempted to take over this natural process, which is known as the medicalisation of menopause. Management of menopause benefits from appropriate medical assessment, including mental and emotional factors as well as the physical. Menopause is neither a medical nor a mental condition, but a natural stage in life that all women go through, although it may be associated with medical problems. About 50 percent of women have no physical or emotional trouble at all. However, many women do need emotional support and counselling, but they are not being heard, nor are they having their questions answered.

We all change and we all go through many changes, but for many women 'the change' (i.e. the menopause) is a time of huge significance. For some women it is just another step on the journey, marked only by the calendar and the absence of periods. For a small minority it is almost a death before death, with sweeping changes, both physical and emotional, which are barely tolerable. Virginia Woolf asked the question: 'Why is life so tragic, so like a strip of pavement over the abyss? I look down: I feel giddy: I wonder how I am ever able to walk to the end.' She suffered from depression for most of her life, but this became untenable around menopause and she finally took her own life. It was a long-standing inner (endogenous) depression related to childhood and teenage distress.

For most women menopause doesn't have to be as overwhelming as Virginia Woolf's experience, but there may be similar long-standing psychological distress that has been covered over or ignored. In fact, it is often the women who have coped and managed to keep at bay the little 'life messages' and 'taps on the shoulder' that have happened through the years who have quite a stockpile of issues waiting to be dealt with at this very important time. Midlife vulnerability tends to expose this. We have seen some women start a new life and others lose their way altogether at menopause, and it is too easy to blame everything on our hormones.

Another frequently asked question is 'When does menopause start?' The usual age is between 45 and 55. The average age of menopause (which is when the last period occurs) is 52, but at whatever age periods cease, twelve months with no periods must elapse before we can call this the last period. However, younger women in their mid-thirties and forties who are still menstruating may note physical and emotional changes that they think could be early menopause though by definition it is not. This is also discussed in later chapters.

Hormone deficiency is only one aspect of menopause; therefore,

HRT is only one aspect of management. Other medical conditions may need to be defined and treated. If the main problem is emotional, women need a sympathetic hearing, some need psychological help and others may need psychiatric treatment. In the last century some women literally went mad at this time of life and were admitted to lunatic asylums. 'A cup of tea, a Bex and a good lie down' (a well known ad on Australian radio in the 1940s and 50s) was often all that was available for our mothers or grandmothers. But to merely cover up the symptoms is no longer adequate, and it was then positively dangerous (long-term use of the phenacetin in Bex tablets caused kidney failure, and these were the days before dialysis and kidney transplants). In the next decade many women were prescribed and became addicted to Valium or Serepax. This became the crutch that they could not throw away.

So if it is not my hormones, is it ME? What is happening to me? What can I do? Most of us now believe that what goes on inside our mind will eventually show up in our body. We are familiar with phrases like 'It makes me sick just thinking about it'; 'Her resentment was eating away at her'; 'He's a real pain in the neck'. We know instinctively that a healthy mind is necessary for a healthy body. Medical research confirms this. But as well as physical and hormonal changes there are emotional responses that can threaten to overwhelm us. If these are understood and dealt with we need not feel helpless. Later we will look at attitudes and perception, about how we see others and ourselves, and examine our behaviour and the choices we make.

We seem to be more aware these days that we are all connected; we are always in relationship to someone or something. This is particularly true for midlife women with children growing up and parents ageing and dying. The choices we make about our own wellbeing will therefore impact on the lives of others as well as on our own lives.

We all want happiness, health and peace of mind, but many women experience instead suffering, loneliness and separation. In underdeveloped countries where women face terror and destruction they undergo constrictions and mutilations that we hear of, but can only barely imagine. Equally there are constrictions and mutilations of the psyche in our 'more enlightened' society which prevent women from enjoying freedom and happiness. The stories in this book may help some women to take away the emotional 'shield' that hides them. All of us want to be happy, and most of us long for inner peace, particularly at midlife when hormonal and emotional changes may bring turmoil.

The following chapters include information and tools that can improve physical and emotional wellbeing for women in midlife as well as stories of women and their journeys to find peace. In our everyday lives and as women in relationships we need ways to help us achieve health and happiness. The theme of practical forgiveness threads its way through the pages that follow, because this is a rich resource for personal liberation, if only we have the willingness to put it into practice.

Part 1

Is it me or my hormones?

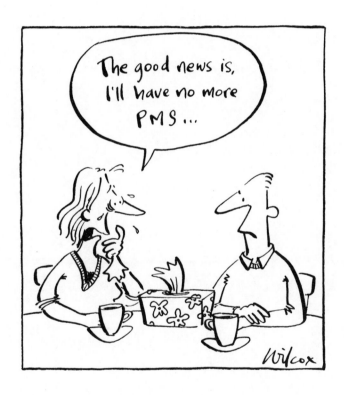

1

Hormones – can we do without them?

If the changes we fear be thus irresistible
What remains but to acquiesce in silence?

Samuel Johnson (1709–1784)

Can we do without hormones? Is menopause an estrogen-deficiency disease, as some doctors claim, requiring hormone replacement therapy for *every* woman, or is it a perfectly natural transition like menarche (the beginning of menstruation), perhaps implying that *no* woman requires HRT?

The word 'hormone' is derived from a Greek word meaning 'setting in motion' or 'messenger'. Sex hormones are *steroid* molecules produced in special glands, mainly the adrenals, ovaries and testes. These hormones are secreted into the bloodstream and travel in the bloodstream to those organs which are able to use them. They are taken up, in certain tissues, by means of *receptors* on the surface of cells. So hormones affect *only* those cells that can take them up. This is different from many other types of medication in common usage, for example, synthetic drugs used to treat high blood pressure, which are less discriminate in their action and may therefore have significant side effects as they act generally in the body not just in the cells which have specific receptors.

Hormones have *specific* actions in *specific* tissues and thus set in motion *specific* responses, such as the growth and division of cells by estrogens and production of nourishing secretions by progesterone.

In this book the word 'hormones' is used to refer to the *female* sex hormones unless otherwise indicated. Note that when the word 'steroid' is used it does not mean 'cortico-steroid', which is the name for powerful hormones produced by the adrenal cortex. Cortico-steroids have acquired a reputation for being strong hormones with significant side effects. They can be lifesaving but must be used with care. The pituitary gland, situated under the front part of the brain, has been called 'the conductor of the endocrine or hormone orchestra', since it secretes hormones to stimulate the various hormone-producing glands.

In the normal menstrual cycle, FSH (Follicle Stimulating Hormone) and estrogen levels start rising as menstruation begins, so we always call the first day of a period the first day of a new cycle. The FSH stimulates several follicles in the ovary to produce estrogens, estradiol being the main estrogen produced. Usually only one follicle becomes the major producer of hormones; the others just fade away. When estrogen levels reach a certain peak, the LH (luteinising hormone) is released from the pituitary gland to stimulate ovulation. If this happens, the egg is released (ovulation) and travels across to the end of the fallopian tube to begin its hopeful journey down to meet the sperm (there are millions of them with, usually, only one winner). Progesterone as well as estrogen is then produced in the follicle and released into the bloodstream to make the body ready for pregnancy. The word 'pro-gest-erone' literally means 'for pregnancy hormone'. If there is no fertilisation, hormone levels drop, the lining of the uterus (endometrium) breaks down, menstruation begins and thus a new cycle starts.

At menopause, when all the eggs (ova) are gone, both FSH and LH rise to high levels and remain high because so little estrogen is produced that there is no feedback to the pituitary to switch off these stimulating hormones. Menstruation ceases because there is now little stimulation of the endometrium and thus no tissue to bleed.

Measurement of estradiol and FSH can therefore help to diagnose menopause. Estradiol will be low and FSH high.

Diagrams of a normal menstrual cycle and the hormone changes in the perimenopausal 'cycle' are included below. The latter is sometimes anything but a cycle, as bleeding may be heavy or light and the period may come sooner or later than the normal 28-day cycle.

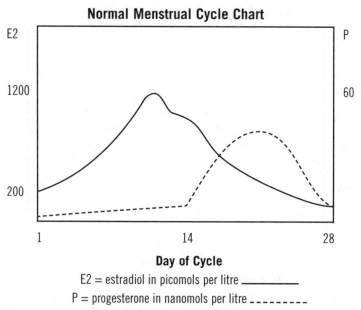

Normal Menstrual Cycle Chart

Day of Cycle

E2 = estradiol in picomols per litre _____

P = progesterone in nanomols per litre _ _ _ _ _ _ _ _

Estrogen

The first day of menstruation is day 1 of a cycle.

In response to FSH (follicle stimulating hormone) from the pituitary gland, estrogens are produced in the follicle of the ovary and estrogen levels rise steadily to mid-cycle, day 14. There is then a small drop in estrogens, they rise again for a few days, and then fall from about day 25. At day 28 levels are below a threshold and the next period starts.

Of course, if conception has occurred, the estrogens continue to rise and pregnancy then switches off the periods for at least nine months.

Progesterone

The progesterone level is low for the first half of the cycle. If ovulation occurs, in response to the LH (luteinising hormone) from the pituitary, then the follicle sheds its egg (ovulation) and the remaining follicle bed secretes progesterone. The level of progesterone rises and then starts to fall about day 25 – when estrogen also falls.

The withdrawal of both the hormones induces the withdrawal bleed that we call the menstrual period, or menstruation.

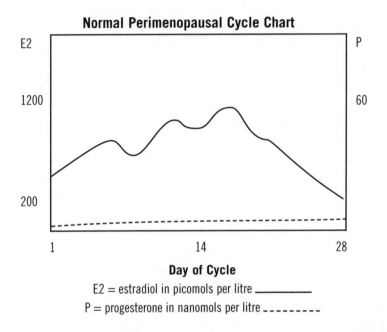

Normal Perimenopausal Cycle Chart

E2 = estradiol in picomols per litre ——————
P = progesterone in nanomols per litre - - - - - - - -

If estrogen levels are high, symptoms such as breast soreness and mood swings may occur. If estrogen levels are low, symptoms of estrogen deficiency such as hot flushes, tiredness and sleep changes may occur, often intermittently.

As show in the figure above, the estrogen levels vary widely and the progesterone level is low for the whole time, as ovulation has not occurred. The lack of progesterone does not, by itself, cause any particular symptoms. Women are at the mercy of their estrogens!

Does this mean that hormones are produced only for reproduction, so that women at the end of reproduction are left high and dry without hormones? This seems rather unfair. Has nature got it wrong? And, even more importantly, *can we do without hormones*? This raises the question we asked at the beginning of the chapter: is menopause an estrogen-deficiency disease or is it a perfectly natural transition?

There is considerable variation in the manifestations of menopause in individual women. The ideal management of the menopausal woman is by *individual assessment*, which should take into account the benefits and risks of treatment or no treatment. Women have said to us that they are afraid of HRT because it is 'chemical and can cause damage to tissues'. In fact, the hormones used these days, although produced in a laboratory, are biologically the same as the estrogens that women themselves produce, so they are not 'chemicals' foreign to the body, unlike most of the pharmaceuticals that are used in modern medicine. Nevertheless, it seems wise to keep doses as low as possible to avoid side effects. Professor Susan Davis from the Jean Hailes Centre in Melbourne recently made a plea in a doctor's magazine to 'Stop bombarding women with HRT'. She suggests that low doses of estradiol administered via a transdermal patch – one which is applied to the skin – is preferable to high doses given orally.

When estrogens are taken by the mouth, they are absorbed by the gut and then processed by the liver. The liver produces a substance called sex-hormone-binding globulin (SHBG), which binds the hormone for transport through the bloodstream. It binds both estrogen and the male hormone testosterone, so high doses of estrogen will push up the SHBG and bind the testosterone that the woman is still producing, thus reducing

Many women can live happy, healthy lives without hormones.

its effectiveness. It is useful to measure testosterone levels in postmenopausal women, particularly if they complain of low libido and lack of energy despite adequate estrogen replacement. I am not saying that all women or even many women need testosterone replacement, just that it is worth considering if libido is low and testosterone levels are low. This will be discussed more fully in Chapter 21. High doses of estrogen *can* cause overactivity of cells: for example, soreness and lumpiness in the breasts may result in some women and we have always to balance the dosage of HRT against possible side effects. My colleague, Dr Barry Wren, says: 'But hormones don't harm tissues; they simply increase the activity of cell function, which is growth and division. So in this sense they have not been proven to cause cancer, but will certainly make estrogen-sensitive cancers grow more rapidly.'

Many women can live happy, healthy lives without hormones. Some women have only a gradual loss of hormones at menopause and no symptoms of their deficiency; it may be that these women produce enough estrogen in their adrenal glands to tide them over. The estrogen referred to here is called *estrone* (which is the hormone used in some HRT, e.g. Premarin and Ogen). Patches, implants and some tablets contain *estradiol*, the main estrogen produced in the ovaries during reproductive life. Thus estrone and estradiol are natural in the real sense.

Some women cope with mild to moderate symptoms easily or prefer not to seek help. Others may avoid hormone therapy despite experiencing symptoms of menopause because of personal factors such as a high risk of clotting or recent breast cancer. Women need sufficient information to help them make the choice whether or not to take hormone replacements.

Some women prefer to use what they call 'natural' products such as soy derivatives and certain herbs (e.g. black cohosh, ginseng, etc.). Although some of these are called plant estrogens, they are not the same as women's own estrogens and thus are not very effective in relieving true estrogen-deficiency symptoms. They are often more expensive than HRT and unfortunately have not undergone rigorous scientific trials.

Summary

- Menopause is a natural event.
- Some women pass through it uneventfully; some women have symptoms due to hormone deficiency and need hormone treatment.
- Women need individual assessment to decide the benefits and risks of hormone therapy.
- Natural products (usually not real hormones) are available but have not undergone scientific trials.

2

What else is happening in midlife?

Nothing is certain but uncertainty.

Latin proverb

Is everything that happens during midlife and menopause merely a reflection of our hormonal state? What else is happening? A lot may be happening, often too much for a woman (or those around her) to cope with. Despite labour-saving devices, many women are busier than ever before and certainly busier than their mothers were. Family problems are different, with relationships and marriages breaking down, and children on drugs or jobless.

Gail's story gives us an idea of the types of issues that may be confronting the menopausal or postmenopausal woman.

It's all happening!

Gail is 60. She had a relatively late menopause. Her periods ceased at age 54 and she had classic symptoms for which she was given HRT, with good results. She stopped this after three years because she felt she did not need it and she was also having breast soreness and gaining weight. She is now tired and is not sleeping well. She has some palpitations and is not coping with day-to-day events.

Her doctor suggested that she go back on HRT, but she is concerned about the risk of breast cancer, particularly because her mother had this type of cancer. This occurred at a late age and her mother died of heart failure, not breast cancer. Though this may not increase Gail's own risk, it certainly makes her more wary of taking HRT.

Gail is clinically depressed. It is mild, but she has the classic symptom of early morning wakening. She described herself this way: 'I don't feel hopeless, but I feel copeless!' All her life she has coped well even though there has been much to test her. When we went through her family situation there was enough there to make anyone want to give up! Her eldest son is an alcoholic and has left his marriage and two small children. Her daughter has been on drugs. Her youngest son has had a life-threatening cancer. Her husband was more and more absent from home, supposedly on business, and then came home and was behaving so oddly that she had to tackle him about it. He finally admitted that he was involved with another woman and that he wanted a divorce so that he could remarry. Within the next six months her sister divorced her husband after 30 years of marriage, their father died and her younger sister, aged 50, died of cancer.

The question 'What else is happening?' is very relevant here. This is a situation where the loss of hormones is no longer causing physical symptoms. Gail went through the stage of hot flushes and these were relieved by HRT at that time. Her present depression is caused mainly by outside circumstances. This is called *exogenous*, or outside, *depression*, as opposed to *endogenous depression*, which comes from something within and may be biochemical. Gail's is an emotional rather than a physical problem. She does not need HRT, or antidepressants, but she *does* need to be listened to and have her grief and loss validated. She also needs to be shown a way to change her attitude. It is possible to choose what happens rather than feel that things just 'happen' to us. At times like this women need to support each other: close friendships can be lifesaving and support groups can be helpful.

Medicalisation of menopause is a stumbling block for many women, particularly with the adverse and contradictory publicity given to recent research data on HRT. However, we can't afford to use this as a reason to go back into the 'dark ages' and pretend nothing is happening.

As discussed in many of the following chapters, there are so many things happening to women at this stage and they all seem to be colliding in the corridor called 'midlife'. The aches, pains and limitations of the ageing body are quite natural, and while these can certainly be improved with exercise, diet, attitude and lifestyle, somewhere in the midst of this comes the realisation that life is very short and our time here is limited. If 'this is as good as it gets' we had better find constructive ways to make the most of it.

Take charge of your choices

Whether we feel fear-based emotions or those that make us peaceful inside is really a matter of choice. Most of us probably don't realise the extent to which we are constantly making choices minute by minute every day. As a woman in midlife you may have to face a number of critical life events and, as a result, you will have choices to make in how you respond:

- Your parents may become very frail and need your emotional and physical help.
- You will probably go through the death of your parents.
- You may experience the death of someone you love.
- You or your husband, or both, may be made redundant and have to face a change of career and life circumstance.
- Your marriage or relationship may falter or break.
- One of your children may get involved in drug or alcohol abuse.

- Children may leave to get married or to live in another country.
- You may be asked to look after grandchildren when you are trying to work full time yourself or have just retired and are planning to travel. This may happen because one of your children is suffering from drug abuse, illness, death of a partner or a marriage break-up.
- One of your children may 'come out'.

The things listed above are all 'life events', not mistakes or something that goes wrong. Some people have more difficulty than others when something knocks them off their tracks. It is often those who have coped well with everything all their lives who experience the most distress. Those women who have managed to get busy and 'get on with it' up till now may feel defeated when things appear 'out of control'.

The cessation of periods is not the only 'change' that happens at midlife. It is a time of many, many changes.

The cessation of periods is not the only 'change' that happens at midlife. It is a time of many, many changes. Very few of these changes give us *choice* over whether they will or won't happen. What we do have, though, is total choice about how we *respond* to these life changes. We are the maestros and conductors of our attitudes. It is our attitude that will determine how we see and experience these changes.

Victor Frankl, a Jewish psychiatrist imprisoned in Auschwitz during World War II, experienced the wiping out of most of his family. He wrote a book called *Man's Search for Meaning* on his observations of human behaviour during this unimaginably horrendous time in our history. His is a memorable quote about attitude and choice: 'The last of the human freedoms is to choose one's *attitude*; to choose one's way'.

Frankl observed that people who responded, even in these atrocious circumstances, from love-based attitudes (sharing meagre resources, helping others) survived physically, emotionally and spiritually more intact, while those who reacted from fear-based emotions and attitudes fared less well, both at that time and later after the war. We can only feel gratitude to a man like this who, despite his suffering, has given us a wonderful legacy to apply to our own lives.

One of the greatest changes for good we can ever make in our lives is a shift from a reliance on fear-based emotions to a commitment and trust in love-based emotions and attitudes. It is a certain formula for inner peace. It is said that our brain functions optimally when we feel safe, yet most of us were raised on fear-based emotions such as:

- Fear of punishment – 'If you don't sit still look out.'
- Fear of failure – 'You call that a report card, I'm really disappointed in you.'
- Fear of loss of love – 'How could you do this, I don't know what to think about you.'
- Fear of abandonment – 'If you are not dressed, young lady, by the time I count to three, I'm leaving this house without you.'

Is any of this familiar to you, either as a child or as a parent? We are all so programmed with fear that we carry it in every cell of our body. We therefore face the challenge of learning to breathe *safety* back into our body, our mind and our heart. Fear impedes higher thinking and keeps us focused on what we can't do, or how hard it is, or how bad it will be if we fail.

A young friend, after obtaining his driver's licence, decided to take an advanced Defensive Driving School course run by the police department. One of the things he had to do, as part of the course, was drive straight at three witch's hats, brake, and then swerve around them without hitting them. Each time he tried, he hit at least one of the hats. The instructor then told him *not* to focus on the witch's hats, but to focus on the *space* where he wanted to go. It then became quite simple to miss the hats and complete the obstacle course.

There is a wonderful saying: 'What you worry about will come about. Please focus on vision.' If you keep your focus on how bad things are, you inevitably end up feeling inadequate for whatever you need to handle. There will be an unwillingness to try to deal with painful situations or difficulties. There will also be that little voice gnawing away saying you can't manage, or you will fail, or it's all too hard. This creates stress reactions in your body, stimulating *old* fear feelings from the past carried to the brain by the limbic system, which will most certainly play havoc with your hormones.

It can be quite devastating when a number of issues start colliding in the corridors of midlife. It really does help to know you have a choice. It helps to create safety so that you don't feel backed into a corner. Making a choice removes you from the role of victim. Victor Frankl couldn't change his circumstances, but he did take power over his attitude. In that sense, he was not a victim. **We may not always be able to change the situation in which we find ourselves, but we most certainly do have choice about the attitude and feelings we bring to the situation.**

We may not always be able to change the situation in which we find ourselves, but we most certainly do have choice about the attitude and feelings we bring to the situation.

I can see how my own attitudes and feelings about others keep me separate from them and may cause pain for me and for those around me. It helps me to pin little cards on the fridge, the bathroom mirror, the car dashboard etc. to remind me that I can choose what I feel at a particular moment. Some that help me are:

- I can choose peace instead of this.
- Do I want to be right or do I want to be happy?
- To be peaceful is merely to focus full attention on it.
- The only person you can change is you.
- Focus on the things that connect you, not the differences.

It helps to have simple daily tools that reinforce and remind you that you have free will and choice hourly and daily. The most immediate thing is your language: the words you use, either silently in your head or with others, are all data for the brain's computer. You may hear yourself saying, 'I have to exercise' or 'I should phone Judy'. But you don't have to. These are choices. You could just as easily say 'I *am* going to exercise' or 'I *will* phone Judy'. Language is extremely powerful and sends continual messages and programming to the brain.

It's very difficult not to blame others for how we feel. Our *own* attitudes, perceptions and thoughts cause our distress, not *other* people, events or things. I know with absolute certainty that this statement is true, but it is so hard to really believe it when I am in the thick of things. It is also apparent in Tessa's story.

Tessa was the matriarch of a large prominent Italian family, whose life had completely fallen apart because of her son. There were four children in her family. A daughter, a lawyer, was now married and had had her first baby. Her oldest son was a successful businessman and the second son was in the family business. Where this woman had come undone was around her youngest son, Anthony. Tessa described Anthony as the brightest and most intelligent of all her children. He had obtained a very high score at the end of secondary school and had enrolled in engineering at university. Midway through the first year he dropped out and became involved with what Tessa called 'a strange bunch of people who led him astray'.

When he was 20 he told his parents that he was homosexual and they threw him out of the family home. Six years later, Tessa was in a total state of trauma, guilt and depression. She said, 'I wish he could have cancer or some ordinary thing that people would understand.' She had removed herself from her circle of friends because, she said, 'they will ask me how Anthony is, and I won't know what to say'. Only immediate family members knew that Anthony was gay. She would not go to extended family weddings and parties because 'they will ask me what he is doing, or if he has a girlfriend'.

Tessa's whole life as she had known it had crumbled. She could not sleep and was.on medication both day and night for her panic attacks, anxiety and depression. She was living in total fear that some person would find out her son was gay. She found it almost impossible to see that Anthony was not the cause of her problems. 'If he would just get himself a girlfriend and a good job I would be well again', she used to say. This was a very good learning experience for me, too, because it was so obvious that blame was keeping Tessa an emotional, physical and spiritual cripple. By believing that Anthony was the cause of her problems she had effectively put him in charge of her wellbeing. She had given her power of free will away. In giving away the power of free will, what followed was a feeling of total helplessness and worthlessness.

Tessa's reactions and responses make it very clear that our ability to make choices and take responsibility for those choices is a measure of self-esteem. Equally, the more blame, the less self-worth.

Tessa became alienated from her world and her friends, the family she loved and herself. With gentle, step-by-step encouragement Tessa was helped to face her guilt, her shame and her fear of judgement. She slowly entered a process of self-forgiveness. Then, with great courage, she told her mother about Anthony and how scared she had been of upsetting her mother and of being judged. She told her about how alone and trapped in silence she had been for the past seven years and what it had done to her health. Her mother held her and they both cried and asked forgiveness of each other.

A month or so later, Tessa and her husband both went to see Anthony to ask his forgiveness for their judgement. Over the following months they talked, cried, shared and loved each other. He was invited home to family meals and gradually his partner was made welcome too. On Anthony's birthday a year later they invited him to have a family party in their home and invite along some of his friends.

Tessa is a warm, compassionate and caring woman. She has taken back her place in her family and community and is a wonderful power for good. When she speaks with warm, reassuring eyes, you know she is coming from the authority and wisdom of a soul who has travelled the road of life's experience.

One of the greatest steps you can take towards freedom and happiness is to take charge of your choices. When you realise the power is within you to be happy, that it does not come from your ability to convince or manipulate others, you can become a conscious choice-maker, or you can be controlling – it's up to you. One choice leads to high self-esteem and inner peace; the other to frustration and powerlessness. *The only person you can change is you.*

Summary

- Many different things are happening to women at midlife, so it is important to identify those symptoms that are due to hormone deficiency.
- Many symptoms have an emotional basis.
- We do have choices; our attitudes may cause our distress rather than other people or events.
- The only person you can change is you.

3

If it's not menopause, what is it?

Ask no questions and you will be told no lies.

18th century proverb

Many women complain that they ask the question, 'If it's not menopause, what is it?', and are fobbed off with a non-committal and generally unhelpful reply, 'Well, it's not menopause.' No alternative answer is offered. Many women at midlife feel that they are not given answers because their question is either not understood or it is disregarded. Perhaps there is no easy answer. It is possible that a woman is going in and out of menopause, so measuring hormones on more than one occasion may provide an answer.

If a woman is still having menstrual periods, then, by strict definition, she is not menopausal. Thus, measuring hormone levels may not say anything except that it is *not* truly menopause because the estrogen levels are still normal, at least on this occasion.

A woman can expect to have this explained to her and be told that she is *perimenopausal*. This tells her that she is going in and out of menopause and therefore is likely to be feeling rather confused about where she is hormonally. For some women, hot flushes, tiredness and other classic symptoms of menopause may occur intermittently, even before periods cease altogether. Measuring hormones several times within a cycle may show marked drops in estrogen hormones, proving that the symptoms *are* heralding menopause and, if the symptoms are severe, that she may need estrogen treatment. However, there is a general reluctance to treat a woman with hormones if she is still menstruating. Hormone treatment given before periods have completely ceased may lead to some bleeding irregularities, but this can usually be worked out satisfactorily. We need not withhold hormone therapy because a woman is still menstruating, but it can be tricky to get the dose right, without causing side effects, such as sore breasts, when the woman's own hormones are kicking in for part of the cycle.

If the menstrual periods are normal and specific symptoms occur just before a period, this may be the so-called *premenstrual syndrome* (PMS) rather than menopause. The symptoms in this case are more likely to be due to high or unbalanced hormones rather than lack of estrogen and are therefore the opposite of the estrogen-deficiency menopause symptoms. These symptoms are breast soreness, bloating and irritable moods (rather than the flushes and sleep disturbance, which are so characteristic of menopause). But some women have a mixture of all these symptoms. It needs careful sorting out: a woman's symptoms may be more important than her hormone levels.

The five cardinal symptoms of menopause are:

- cessation of periods
- hot flushes (plus or minus sweats)
- a change in sleep pattern
- a feeling of ants crawling under the skin
- a dry vagina.

We can add anxiety/panic attacks, if these have occurred at menopause and there has been no other obvious cause.

These symptoms are most *directly* related to hormone deficiency, and to estrogen deficiency, in particular. There are very many others listed in various books and pamphlets, but most are less specific than these five.

It must be said clearly at this point that *the main cause of the symptoms that occur at menopause is estrogen deficiency.* Progesterone, our other female hormone, is only present for half of the menstrual cycle and, close to menopause, is absent most of the time since it depends on ovulation to produce it and ovulation is infrequent at this stage of life (i.e. women are infertile). So the absence of progesterone does not cause any major symptoms, whereas the absence of estrogen does. This contradicts the claims of progesterone protagonists who have taken up the work of Dr John Lee, an American physician who has written many books for lay people. He claims that before and after menopause progesterone deficiency is more important so that progesterone replacement can be used *instead* of estrogen. He recommends the use of natural progesterone as a cream. However, in a small study conducted by my colleagues and me five years ago, we were unable to reproduce his results.

... there are many symptoms that are menopause-like, such as tiredness, lack of libido, aches and pains, depression etc., which may have other causes

It is also important to understand that there are many symptoms that are menopause-like, such as tiredness, lack of libido, aches and pains, depression etc., which may have other causes. In medical terms, we need to make a *differential diagnosis*, i.e. we need to look for other medical causes of the symptoms. Here are some of the other conditions which may occur at this time and cause confusion:

- *Anaemia* and decreased iron levels will cause tiredness. There will usually be a history of heavy blood loss in the perimenopause to account for this or it may be related to diet, particularly strict vegetarianism.
- *Decreased thyroid* production will cause tiredness, dry skin, weight gain and perhaps loss of libido.
- *Increased thyroid* production will cause anxiety, palpitations,

sleep disturbance, weight loss, and feeling hot rather than having flushes, sometimes known as 'global warming'.

- *Liver disease* may cause tiredness, though usually acute viral hepatitis has jaundice as the obvious sign.
- Some rare conditions related to other hormones cause sweating with or without flushing (see Madeleine's story on page 33).
- *Depression*, and the drugs used to treat it, can cause sleep disturbance and tiredness.
- *Sleep apnoea* can be a cause of tiredness. This condition, which occurs in men as often as in women, is usually associated with snoring. Breathing becomes irregular and shallow. Oxygen intake decreases. The sufferer wakes in the morning having slept apparently deeply, but still feeling tired.
- Serious illnesses such as *cancer* may be present, causing tiredness, aches and pains, and many other vague symptoms.

Other disorders that may appear, such as arthritis, mild diabetes and increased blood pressure, are more related to ageing than to hormone deficiency. These cause other symptoms rather than those typical of menopause.

It is important that we do not ascribe all symptoms that occur at this time to hormone deficiency. But it is also important to recognise that, for *some* women, estrogen deficiency, by itself, may cause *severe* symptoms. This is especially true for younger women who have had both ovaries removed and thus have had an early surgical menopause, what we sometimes call a 'crash' menopause. Going from high hormone levels to almost none within a few hours is catastrophic. Women who have had a hysterectomy, but still have one or both ovaries, may find it hard to tell when they reach menopause since they don't have periods anyway. Measuring hormones is the only way to be sure. If both ovaries are removed at the time of the hysterectomy the woman is truly postmenopausal.

Women who are still on the oral contraceptive pill at midlife find it difficult to know whether they have reached menopause or have gone through it. The only way to tell is to stop taking the pill and then have hormone levels checked a few weeks later. (It is advisable to use alternative contraception until you are sure that menopause has been reached. The chance of getting pregnant is very small but miracles/accidents do happen.)

Menopause occurring before the age of 40 is called 'premature'. In some cases, this is only temporary because the ovaries may cease functioning for months or even years, but then respond again for a while. Blood tests are needed to work out what is happening. Severe stress may also play a causal role in stopping periods. The appropriate blood tests are estradiol (estrogen), which falls markedly, and FSH (or follicle stimulating hormone), produced by the pituitary gland, which rises to a persistently high level if a woman is truly menopausal, as we have seen in Chapter 1.

The *perimenopause* is a period of months or years before the menopause when the menstrual cycle begins to change. Bleeding may become very heavy or light, and hot flushes may come and go, sometimes interspersed with PMS-type symptoms such as breast soreness and mood swings. It can be truly a roller-coaster ride for some unfortunate women (and their partners and families) (see Chapter 10). Blood tests once or twice monthly at critical times may be the only way to determine what is happening. Some women may be menopausal one month and ovulating the next. Most are able to cope with the ups and downs of this phase of life if someone can help them understand what is happening.

So, is it you or your hormones? It may well be both, or it may be something else altogether, such as a general medical illness or an emotional crisis.

Julie was aged 36 when she had her tubes tied. The gynaecologist was surprised to find only one ovary present though she had no history of previous removal of an ovary. At the age of 38 her menstrual cycle faltered and she had such severe night sweats that changing the bedclothes became a nightly occurrence. She also suffered sleep disturbance and mild depression. She was given HRT, which suppressed the night sweats, but her bleeding pattern was now unpredictable. She was referred to me because of the bleeding 'problem'. Further questioning revealed that in the two previous months she had had bleeding a month apart, preceded by breast soreness and mood swings (up rather than down). This all sounded classically premenstrual. She stopped the HRT and felt normal. Blood tests revealed that she was not yet menopausal.

Is she or is she not menopausal? Yes and no. She may slip back into a more regular pattern for some months but is probably heading for an early menopause. Her mother ceased her periods at about 42. What else may be causing this? Julie's social and family history revealed some stressful elements, which may be contributing to her present menstrual chaos. We know that severe life-threatening situations such as serious illness, starvation weight loss, or death of a close one may cause cessation of periods, but the role of lesser stresses is less clear.

Julie married at 18 'a man who was able to handle my mother', as she put it. Her mother was dominating and emotionally violent. She did not show love physically to any of her children (she had not received love as she grew up).

Julie has three older brothers. She also has an all-male household of three sons. Her husband, Maurice, is a controller and she is not sure whether she wants to stay in the marriage. While overseas recently, he sent her a nine-page fax explaining why he was leaving permanently and what was wrong with her. To her surprise and dismay, he then came home as if nothing had happened. They have recently moved house. Her middle son has mild ADD and needs extra attention. The six-year-old much-loved family dog became ill and she nursed it. Her sons could not cope with the dog's illness so she had to do this alone. It was expensive financially as well as emotionally. She and Maurice have recently attended counselling sessions. Julie feels angry and distressed that the sessions do not seem to do much except encourage confrontation. She says that she and Maurice are still trying to cope as a couple with the skills that they had at 18 and these are no longer adequate or helpful.

So if it's not menopause, what will help? Medically it is best to wait and see, i.e. not to give hormones but to measure hormone levels. If periods cease and symptoms return, then appropriate HRT may be the answer. Emotionally, Julie needs help. She is angry. She feels unheard. She needs to decide what is best for her. If Maurice is not willing to change, and does not see the need to, can she cope and find a way to validate herself? Does she need to leave the marriage? She needed some help to decide this, so I sent her to see Patricia who now takes up the story:

To some degree we all use denial as a coping tool. Whenever life presents us with a difficult or painful situation we have a tendency to create a more palatable fantasy. At this time it has a lifesaving and protective function, i.e. how we learned to cope and survive as children. When things were tough we just got on with life and did the best we could.

Julie certainly did this in finding a 'knight in shining armour' to whisk her away from her mother and to stand up and do battle for her. Unfortunately for Julie, the *dragon slayer* turned into the *dragon*. Her husband, Maurice, became more and more like her mother. This seemed so strange to Julie. How could it be? The more she tried to avoid dealing with this part of herself (the part controlled by her mother and now by her husband) the stronger it became. At one level, of course, forgetting about unpleasant things in our childhood appears to work. We survive, don't we? And that is not to be sneezed at. But these unresolved issues don't go away. They lie deep within us, and then surface in all sorts of ways, sometimes when we least expect it. They often confront us in the people closest to us. It's as if life is willing to keep giving us fresh opportunities to get rid of the junk that clutters our heads. In Julie's case, it was her relationship with her husband that stirred buried junk.

In many ways Julie never had a model to show her 'how to be a woman', or a responsible adult. She became the third generation of women in the family not to receive warmth and affection. As a consequence she was too timid and afraid to stand up for herself and fight her own battles. She longed for someone to look after her and care for her. As the only girl in her family she was quite sheltered and protected and was never encouraged to be strong and self-reliant. At eighteen, Julie handed over to her husband the responsibility for standing up to her mother.

The soothing balm of companionship and protection, which pulled her to her husband, soon turned into the possessive and controlling demands that she had fled from in her mother. It was as if she had been caught in her own snare.

When they went to couples counselling Julie again wanted me to take responsibility and 'save' her from her controlling husband in the same way she had wanted her husband to save her from her controlling mother. In fact, she became quite angry with me when I declined this invitation and began coaching Julie to stand up for herself with her husband. In her despair she had begun to use negative tactics to try to force Maurice to be more loving. She withheld affection by becoming emotionally distant and critical. Julie was encouraged to express all the anger and repressed feelings she held towards her mother.

She was coached and encouraged to relax into feeling at home with herself and shown how to take back the responsibility for her happiness that she had handed over to her husband. Julie and Maurice together were taught how to listen to each other and to begin to respect each other's differences. In learning to listen to each other they created safety in their relationship. It was only then that they became willing to put real effort into working towards an equal and mature love relationship.

This is a skill that anyone can learn and it is a wonderful tool for any relationship – male/female, children, friends and colleagues.

As mentioned above, the symptoms that a woman is experiencing may be nothing to do with menopause at all. There is a very important message here. Just because a woman is in her forties or early fifties does not mean that everything she experiences is due to her hormones. As Doris Lessing said, 'It had been useful, apparently, for the family's mythology, to have a mother in the menopause.'

Sweats and depression are two symptoms sometimes occurring at midlife that may be due to other causes. One of the most dramatic instances of this that I have ever encountered was with Madeleine.

At age 46, Madeleine said, 'Depression suddenly *fell* on me.' Her description was both graphic and unusual. It was so sudden and severe that she had to be admitted to hospital. She had been feeling unwell and behaving oddly with her family for several months. She was experiencing severe head and neck sweats. She felt out of control, and she described her moods as 'vicious', which was again a most unusual description. Her periods were still regular. She was treated with an antidepressant and some of her symptoms got worse. She said, 'I was out of my tree. I seemed to be someone else.'

Not all her friends were helpful and few were sympathetic. One friend told her that she had no reason to be depressed because 'you have a good husband, great children, a lovely house and no financial worries. Pull yourself together and don't be such a pain!' 'You must be mad', someone else told her. She *felt* mad, and sad, and bad! She became suicidal. The dose of antidepressants was increased and she felt even worse. She was losing weight now and having panic attacks. It was *not* just depression. She had never suffered from depression before and there was certainly no reason now for all these feelings.

Somehow she survived this phase, but then she had chest pains and

was seen by a cardiologist. He listened to her unusual story. When he
checked it, her blood pressure was extremely – dangerously – high.
He tested her urine for catecholamines, which are adrenaline and
noradrenaline derivatives, the so-called 'fight and flight' hormones. Sure
enough, she had these and was found on a CT scan to have a tumour
in her adrenal gland. This tumour was pouring out the hormones that
are normally there to protect us but can wreak havoc if not appropriately
switched off.

In this case, the problem was certainly hormonal. And, of course, it was
other hormones, not her female ones. No wonder she felt taken over
and not herself.

Fortunately, this is an extremely rare condition, but it illustrates how
wary we have to be. If not correctly diagnosed, Madeleine's condition
was potentially fatal.

Hot flushes are very characteristic of menopause, but careful questioning may reveal that the cause may not be hormonal.

Pamela was sent to see me for menopause problems. She said that her
periods were fading out and she was experiencing global warming rather
than hot flushes. She said that rather than having intermittent flushing
she felt generally hot and was losing weight. She did not have any
physical signs of hyperactive thyroid, but her story was unusual, so I
checked her thyroid as well as her female hormones. She was right! She
did have global warming, i.e. her whole body was heated by a very
overactive thyroid. She has now been treated and her thyroid is
behaving normally.

This is another good reminder to be aware, always, that not everything
that happens at menopause is due to female hormones. There are other
things happening.

Tiredness and *fatigue* may be caused by poor sleep or excess physical or mental work. Tiredness is also the major symptom of anaemia and iron deficiency.

Josephine complained of extreme tiredness. All her life she had had heavy periods. She welcomed the end of menstruation. She was sleepy in the daytime and wakeful at night. She had had some flushes so her doctor had prescribed HRT. Her tiredness persisted. I checked her iron levels and found that she was anaemic, with very low iron stores. Iron tablets had been prescribed previously but she always gave up taking them because of the constipation they caused. I prescribed a course of iron injections and her tiredness lifted. These symptoms were not due to hormones, but to simple iron deficiency, and the cause was the heavy periods resulting in blood loss.

Thyroid deficiency or underactivity, as opposed to overactivity in Pamela's case, increases with age, so may occur at the same time as menopause. The classic symptoms are *fatigue* and *dry skin*. These symptoms also occur with estrogen deficiency and, of course, these two things, menopause and thyroid deficiency, may occur together.

Margaret is an academic high flyer who travels nationally and internationally. When she 'hit menopause' she felt that she had been stopped in her tracks. She had been given HRT but her energy did not return, though her hot flushes went away. A blood test revealed very low thyroid levels. She has a condition called Hashimoto's Disease, which is an auto-immune problem. The body produces antibodies against its own thyroid hormone-producing cells. Replacement of her thyroid hormone has given her back her zest for living.

The stories presented in this chapter illustrate that there may be other hormones or conditions to blame for certain menopause-like symptoms and that some of these can be truly life threatening. All women therefore deserve to be fully assessed at midlife to correctly determine the cause of symptoms.

Summary

- The perimenopause is a time of fluctuating changes.
- Many symptoms around this time have causes other than hormonal changes.
- Estrogen deficiency causes specific symptoms.
- Changes in other hormones, e.g. thyroid, may be causing symptoms of menopause.
- Women deserve full assessment at midlife to distinguish between physical and psychological disturbance.

4

Just pull yourself together!

Wee sleekit cowrin timorous beastie,
O what a panic's in thy breastie.

Robbie Burns (1759–1796), 'To a Mouse'

Perhaps the most unthinking and uncaring advice that can be given to anyone, man or woman, at midlife or any other time, is this: 'Oh for goodness sake, just pull yourself together!' It is particularly unwelcome to the sufferer of panic attacks. No-one wants to remain engulfed in such fear and anxiety that, at times, it can feel life threatening.

Palpitations, anxiety and panic attacks are triggered in some women by hormonal changes, especially the drops in estrogen that occur at menopause. Panic and anxiety disorders occur in men as well as women and at times other than menopause. According to the WHO Classification of Mental and Behavioural Disorders (1992), 'Panic disorder [episodic paroxysmal anxiety] is characterised by recurrent attacks of severe anxiety [panic] which are not restricted to any particular situation or set of circumstances and which are therefore unpredictable.'

Symptoms vary but include sudden onset of palpitations, chest pain, dizziness, choking sensations, feelings of unreality. The victim feels that she will go mad or lose control or even die. I have known women who have had to pull off a freeway and then sit shaking and fearful, unable to continue driving. The attacks usually last for minutes only but are frightening. A panic attack is often followed by persistent fear of another attack, which may make it impossible for that person to go to certain places or do certain things.

We recommend the book, *Power over Panic*, by Bronwyn Fox as a practical guide to understanding and managing this disorder which causes so much social distress and can sometimes be life threatening.

Sylvia lives in a coastal town 50 kilometres from the city. Her husband, John, brought her to my office. She is afraid to drive because she has had to pull off the freeway on two occasions. Each time she felt she was going to suffocate and pass out. Her heart was beating very fast; she was sweating and felt nauseated and giddy.

Sylvia is aged 52 and has not had a period for five months. She has flushes and night sweats, but these have not worried her particularly and she had decided not to take HRT but to literally 'sweat it out'. She had increased the soy in her diet and was using some herbal remedies.

Before her marriage 30 years ago Sylvia had suffered from bouts of anxiety and fear that she would not be good enough. After each of her two children she had postnatal depression, which was not diagnosed at the time. On each occasion she was told by her mother-in-law to 'pull yourself together'. John has always been supportive and her own parents, though not overly demonstrative, have also been supportive if not completely understanding.

John has recently had to change jobs. Sylvia is concerned about their financial situation and afraid that they may have to sell their home to buy something smaller and cheaper. Her children have left home but are not yet fully self-supporting.

She is now in a spiral of anxiety. Her doctor has suggested that she undertake antidepressant therapy, but she is afraid to do this and afraid of being labelled as depressed or not coping. She does not feel depressed, just anxious and fearful of another attack. All her life she has been a perfectionist and anxious to please.

I persuaded Sylvia to try HRT but did not claim that this would remove her anxiety. We discussed panic attacks and I assured her that, despite the severity of the symptoms, it was not a life-threatening disorder but an exaggeration of the normal 'fight–flight' response. She was much reassured by this and said that she really had been frightened of dying during an attack. She accepted my suggestion of cognitive therapy and relaxation therapy in addition to the HRT. I saw her a month later. She had had two minor panic attacks but was able to cope mainly because she no longer felt afraid of dying during an attack.

Maria was one of the first women I cared for 20 years ago when I started a menopause clinic. She had never been able to come to the clinic because she was agoraphobic and had not ventured outside her house for four years. I visited her at home. She was depressed, anxious and fearful. At this time I had little experience with psychiatric disorder. Because she was having severe sweats and flushes I persuaded her to take HRT. She had not had a period for four years so I did not need to measure her hormone levels to make the diagnosis of estrogen deficiency. A month later I saw her again. She had ventured outside, but only to her front gate. She was happier and her flushes had been controlled. Her husband felt that it would only be a matter of time before she would venture out beyond the front gate. But his hopes were not fulfilled. Maria stopped taking the HRT after six months and panic overwhelmed her again. She had become convinced that nothing could help her and she was literally paralysed by fear.

I suggested that she consider antidepressant therapy but she was unwilling to try this.

Twenty years on I could now offer Maria management of her condition. There were clues to her problem that I did not then consider. Maria was born in Italy. She grew up in a large hardworking family with little money. She left school in her teens and worked on the family farm. Her mother died of breast cancer when Maria was fifteen, so she helped to rear six younger siblings. When she was twenty-five her father arranged a marriage with an older man. They then migrated to Australia. Maria spoke no English. There was little chance for her to learn. She had five children in the next eight years and worked hard with her husband in their market garden. Her children looked down on her because of her poor English and semi-literacy. As the children grew up and married she became increasingly isolated and had little self-esteem. At menopause she put on weight and felt useless. While shopping one day she had a panic attack. She subsequently refused to go out even though her husband offered to go everywhere with her. Her children all told her to pull herself together. Maria's problem was not just menopausal breakdown but a life process which came to a head in midlife.

The next story gives hope that panic disorder can be helped with understanding, reassurance and therapy, including self-help.

Barbara was 51 when I first met her. She was smartly dressed, slim and intelligent, but her coping skills had deserted her. She had always looked after everyone else – mother, sisters, husband, children – but now she was weeping for no reason, unable to decide what to cook for dinner and besieged by panic attacks when she tried to drive the car. Her husband could not understand the breakdown. He kept telling her to pull herself together. Her periods had ceased at age 50 and she felt very sure that menopause was just a passing phase, a bend in the road, needing nothing extra to get through it. She was sleeping poorly, experiencing many hot flushes, and she felt embarrassed by the sweating which unravelled her usually neat hairdo. But her major distress was the feeling of being unable to cope after a lifetime of *always* coping. Her graphic description of her predicament was: 'I'm like a car without a steering wheel.'

HRT helped the physical symptoms but the emotional mayhem and panic attacks did not respond. I sent her for psychiatric help and she had to be admitted to a private hospital under the care of a psychiatrist. Appropriate antidepressant drugs and psychotherapy over the next three months gradually restored proper functioning.

The lid had to be removed to expose a lifetime of coping with hurt and emotional abuse.

Barbara grew up surrounded by strict family rules and expectations. She was told, 'Don't cry, don't laugh too much or too loudly, always get everything *absolutely* right.' All this was hidden behind her protective perfect façade. Certainly the hormonal upheavals caused some cracks in this mask, but to merely fill in the cracks with HRT would have been to miss the opportunity to deal with the hidden torments and hurts which would have exploded like a volcano down the track.

Some two years later, Barbara stopped both her HRT and her mild antidepressant medication and she turned up again, distressed and angry that she was not cured of her affliction. She had stopped the HRT because she had breast soreness and was concerned about possible breast cancer risk. I explained to her that I believe that hormones do not *cause* breast cancer, but estrogens do make breast cells grow and divide, so may promote the growth of a breast cancer already there and can make breasts active and sometimes painful. Breast soreness does not mean cancer. It simply means that the breasts are very sensitive to the action of estrogens so the dose needs to be kept very low or else estrogens need to be stopped.

Once again she was given anti-anxiety medication and asked to look at her underlying hurts and to continue to deal with them. This time she did not need HRT, just the simple anti-anxiety therapy. In view of her breast sensitivity it was better not to give HRT this time.

Recently, a synthetic compound called tibolone has become available. Developed in the UK around fifteen years ago, it mimics some of the effects of estrogen and testosterone, and so can relieve symptoms like hot flushes, dry vagina and low libido without causing growth of breast tissue or the endometrium (the lining of the uterus). This could have been useful for Barbara but was not available at that time.

So was it Barbara or her hormones? It was *both*, but it was the emotional issues that most needed dealing with at that stage. Patricia spent time with Barbara and was able to help her answer these questions. Here are her comments:

> Barbara's story is an extreme example of a very common occurrence that I often come across in working with women in midlife. But I think it is reflective of a deeper problem expressing itself in society generally.
>
> Most of us are out of touch with who we really are. Our core self gets covered by an adapted self that knows how to please and perform in order to be loved and valued. This adapted self has extra sensory skills and perception that it uses to perfection. In a group of people, or one-on-one, it knows instantly if a bright and breezy conversation is required or a deep and meaningful one is called for. So what it ends up getting is its outside shell being stroked for performance and achievements. It is praised for results and valued for ability to 'do it'; whatever the 'it' may be – to get good grades at school, go to university, have the gym-trimmed body, be the ideal wife, hostess, mother, P & C president – it will deliver. It will do whatever is needed to get the pat on the back in order to feel worthwhile.
>
> The sad thing is that while this adapted performance shell is out there doing, the inside core self remains almost untouched by any of it. It is very lonely and unseen for who it really is. It's almost as if it has lived a lifetime of jumping through hoops in order to be loved and appreciated. But no-one knows who the person really is, nor does she (or he) know. I want to stress here that there is nothing wrong with any

of these very worthwhile endeavours and achievements. In fact, they are all worthy of credit. The problem arises when we become so identified with what we do that we lose touch with who we really are.

The reason we are tired, depressed, frightened and unimaginative is that we are out of touch with our true self. We have forgotten who we really are.

Barbara needed to look very deeply into the expectations that were placed on her by a very critical and demanding mother and an over-competitive father. After a time she could see that her perfectionist drive to be loved and valued by them became a life pattern. The critical words of her mother became an internalised critic inside Barbara's head. This voice drove her on to be a perfectionist in all things, but no matter what she did it was not quite perfect, never enough to satisfy the perfectionist in her head. When she was younger she had the energy to keep driving herself. But now she had lost the will and the way.

Years ago, when I first started a journey of personal growth, phrases like 'one part of me tells me I'm not good enough' or 'I'm giving myself a hard time' were often heard in groups that I attended. They seemed to reflect peoples' experiences, feelings and memories.

The limbic system is the part of the brain that deals with our feelings and memory. As children we develop mechanisms that help us survive situations that are too stressful for us to handle at an early age. In childhood these strategies protect us and help us to cope and survive. Barbara became the perfectionist to protect herself from being criticised by her mother. As adults the painful, stressful memories may be unavailable to conscious awareness but still remain in our nervous system. Our body is constantly 'at the ready', in a continual state of adrenal alert. When this continual alertness is happening outside our awareness it can be very damaging to our physical and emotional health because nature intends us to be in a state of relaxed joyfulness.

Through oceans of tears, Barbara did the healing work necessary to free her from the memory of her mother's expectations. She reached deep inside herself to touch the riches of the human spirit, her True

Self. She found that she no longer craved the outside strokes and praise because she was in touch with the power inside.

Barbara is now vital and happy and once again enjoying her husband's retirement. This change of heart, this awakening, ignited the possibility of life's beauty finding expression with her family and friends. For the first time she felt compassion and appreciation for the one inside who had tried so hard all her life, for the part of herself who had stuck in there with her through thick and thin, never giving up on her. In fact, as Barbara relaxed deeper into the one inside, she discovered moments of deep inner peace and absolute perfection.

As a menopause physician I am grateful to have colleagues who can deal with symptoms not directly caused by hormone deficiency. In each of the three cases presented here, HRT was of some benefit for associated physical symptoms, but the main tools needed were emotional support, understanding and psychotherapy because the main problem was not simply hormones.

Summary

- Panic disorder occurs in men as well as women. It can feel life-threatening.
- Panic disorder at menopause may be related to hormone changes and respond to hormone therapy.
- For women who have breasts which are very sensitive to estrogen, the synthetic compound tibolone, a 'hormone look-alike', may be useful.
- In some cases, psychological or psychiatric treatment may be required.

5

Emotional midlife

No person was ever rightly understood until they had been first regarded with a certain feeling, not of tolerance, but of sympathy.

Thomas Carlyle (1795–1881)

Women at the menopause, who have previously been noted for their coping skills, may feel dismayed when these skills are in disarray. Their confidence begins to evaporate, they question themselves and, of course, they ask the question, 'Is it me or my hormones?' If they are told that it is not menopause (usually on the basis of *one* blood test only), they seek reassurance and are often dismissed or told, 'Just pull yourself together.' Usually their periods are haywire, so they are certainly perimenopausal and further blood tests may show that they are actually going in and out of menopause. In some ways this 'going in and out' is harder to cope with than the true menopause (when periods have ceased for at least six months and classic symptoms have started).

It is so easy to blame *all* that happens around this time on hormones, but it is also too easy to blame the women themselves. These women are asking for understanding and support, not ridicule. Some words sung by Bob Dylan in his song, 'The times they are a-changing', apply here: 'Please don't criticise what you don't understand.'

Jill is in her late forties. She has always been confident and able to deal with things. She has brought up three children, supported Max, her husband, in his business ventures, and has had a career of her own in fashion design. She has elderly parents who are relatively fit physically, but her mother has become forgetful so she needs support in making decisions.

Recently Jill has felt shaky at times, both physically and emotionally. Her periods have become irregular. She may go for two or three months without a period and then have a period that lasts for weeks or else is barely there. She has some flushes and finds herself surprisingly moved to tears, often about things, especially on TV, which would not normally directly concern her. She has been embarrassed at times when she has burst into tears at work for no obvious reason. She feels less confident than she did and cannot imagine how she coped in the past with real family crises.

She and Max go to the same general practitioner, and she has now become incensed by what she calls their 'jokey-blokey behaviour'. When she went to her doctor asking for help for her emotional and physical ups and downs, he just said, 'Well, what can you expect at your age' and joked about her loss of confidence. He even used the well-worn but not reassuring phrases, 'Just pull yourself together' and 'You'll get over it given time.' Her doctor had discussed her symptoms with Max and joked about her lapses in confidence.

When she came to see me she was angry, distressed and confused. 'I am not a silly woman', she said. Jill is far from silly. She is intelligent and well informed. But about this time of life she has been given no information and she thus feels as if something is happening to her control. She has managed a family, a marriage and a career, and suddenly she feels shipwrecked. She is well groomed and capable, but her sudden swings in mood and the embarrassing tears and flushes have undermined her mental confidence. Added to this is the physical tiredness due to sleep disturbance because of night sweats. Her libido is also lower. Her husband is not joking about this, fortunately, but she feels the lack and has some guilt about it (a common female reaction). However, his lack of understanding about her other symptoms does not make her want to rush into his arms. She has a mixture of conflicting emotions, much of which is due to swinging hormones.

Jill is undergoing perimenopause. Her ovaries can no longer respond appropriately to the pituitary-stimulating hormone (FSH). She has few remaining eggs capable of responding, so she is not ovulating. Menopause can be predicted to happen in the next two to three years. Her hormonal swings are also not helping her sexual performance, as feeling hot may make cuddling difficult and low estrogens may reduce sensation and responses. She feels angry with Max for his apparent lack of understanding and concern, so she is inclined to repel his advances. In addition, her male hormone (testosterone) was low when measured, so her libido and orgasmic response have diminished.

What can Jill do? Hormone supplementation may help. By this I mean that, rather than full replacement, smaller doses are given in cyclic fashion – three weeks of hormones with a week's break. Women who tolerate the oral contraceptive pill can use this because it will suppress the unpredictable cycle and give steadiness and predictability. At the same time it will relieve flushes and associated symptoms. Unfortunately, the oral contraceptive pill may not improve libido. The male hormone, testosterone, as a cream or patch, can be used when testosterone levels are very low (see also Chapter 21).

However, in among all these hormonal surges there are swinging emotions as well. Jill feels belittled, misunderstood and lacking in confidence.

So what can she do emotionally? She needs to be validated and supported. She needs to find a more sympathetic and empathetic general practitioner. Most of all, she needs to talk to her husband about her feelings. And this would best be done by a therapist trained in 'couples' therapy so that Max does not feel judged or criticised.

Bridget was a distressed 49-year-old woman when I first saw her at a menopause clinic. Her medical history included rare tropical diseases and, more recently, a viral illness which led to post-viral syndrome, i.e. persistent fatigue (nowadays called Chronic Fatigue Syndrome, or CFS). She had undergone a hysterectomy years earlier so was unsure whether she was menopausal. Her husband had traded her in 'for a much earlier model', as she succinctly put it, so she had brought up her only daughter alone. She had always worked in senior management positions in the hospitality industry so could not understand her present feelings of inadequacy. She showed me her references, which described her abilities in glowing terms. Her own words were graphic: 'I could not believe who I'd now become, given who I had always been, and *I could do nothing about it*. I was not who I used to be. I was living in the shadows.'

Her hormone levels suggested perimenopause rather than menopause. She had been told to pull herself together. No effort on her part had achieved this. Over the next year she became menopausal and HRT was given. This helped her symptoms and she started on the road back to emotional health, though her physical energy took longer to return.

Here is another woman who knew she was not 'a silly woman'. Because of what she went through she has been able to help many others find a way back from lack of self-esteem and despair. For Bridget, hormone deficiency was one factor in her condition but other physical problems were present and these needed different management. Even more importantly, the emotional distress and loneliness she felt kept her in a state of depression. She did not want to take antidepressants and I agreed with her that these were not needed. Reassurance was as important as

Reassurance was as important as the HRT to restore her self-esteem.

the HRT to restore her self-esteem. She had a strong religious faith which had sustained her through many crises. As she became more aware, mostly from her own experience but also by asking for help from those close to her, she felt her depression lift.

Longing for yesterday

Why she had to go I don't know, she didn't say,
I said something wrong, now I long for yesterday.

The Beatles, *Yesterday*

The section of The Beatles' song quoted above suggests that men lament the loss of a partner and are baffled by her departure. As the lack of communication in the relationship becomes obvious, they feel guilt as well as abandonment. Women also have these feelings when the male partner leaves.

Jocelyn was in her mid-fifties when her husband confessed that he had met a younger woman in his acting group and wanted out. Jocelyn was devastated. She had suspected that he was seeing someone else, but did not feel that she could confront him. He had taken a flat close to the city 'to be closer to work during the week'. She had gone around to his flat and had seen the other woman's car there, but she could not talk to him about this. She sold the family home and moved to another suburb. Her self-esteem was rock bottom; she was depressed. She had hung in there even though she knew that he was attracted to other women. This was not the first time that he had left emotionally, if not physically. She hoped that by saying nothing and accepting the situation he would remain with her. She had been chronically ill for much of their married life. He found this very difficult and feared that he would have to look after her in old age just as her father had had to look after her frail mother.

She was going through menopause, but the physical symptoms were not severe enough for her to need HRT. However, she was losing confidence and being deserted was the last straw. She didn't press for divorce and has in fact remained friendly with him, although she would not now have him back. She is still chronically ill and this had been very divisive in the marriage in that she could not keep up with him then, nor can she now. This precipitated her loneliness and deep depression. She struggled emotionally as well as physically.

She was diagnosed with osteoporosis a few years after he left and was put on HRT for this. The HRT helped her moods and general wellbeing as well as her bones. She has now moved into a retirement villa to be near her daughter and family, where she feels useful and wanted.

I asked Patricia to see Jocelyn. These were her comments:

When I first saw Jocelyn she was a frightened, defeated, lonely, sad woman.

As I listened to the story above, it became clear that her problems were not just of her husband's making. In fact, I think that very little of what was happening had its roots in the marriage. The questions that went around inside my head were:

- What was happening inside this woman that she could not bring herself to talk to her husband about what was happening to her – her pain and loneliness and her suspicions about him?
- Where did she learn that to be silent is safe?
- Why was she willing to settle for so little sharing, intimacy and companionship?
- Where did her feelings of shame and lack of worth originate?

I am convinced that humankind's greatest addiction is not to alcohol or drugs but to the emotional addiction of self-doubt. So many of us are deeply convinced that our inherent state is one of worthlessness and inadequacy. This state typically stems from our early childhood and our perception of the events and experiences that we had as a child.

These perceptions, once internalised, colour and shade our whole reality and form a prism through which we view every situation, event and relationship. We need to take time to go inside and heal these early wounds. If we do not, we will continue to re-experience and reinforce our painful beliefs and perceptions.

Jocelyn needed to look at the critical parenting she received as a child. When she was helped to do this, she could see that she was always considered a nuisance if she prevailed upon or interrupted her parents.

She was brought up in the old school of 'children should be seen but not heard', but she never got to be the adult who was both seen and heard. She just replaced her father with her husband. With help and time, Jocelyn was able to look with love and compassion on the young girl of her childhood and see her beauty and strength. She was also able to put into perspective the criticism from her father, who was in his own post-war trauma during a lot of her childhood and adolescence. The pain around her early life had created an obstacle to her feeling loved or worthwhile. For Jocelyn, forgiveness was the undoing of these obstacles and a way to set herself free from the pain she was experiencing. The steps she undertook were to:

- recognise the area of her wounding
- release suppressed emotions
- shed swallowed tears
- let go of the feelings of hurt and shame she was holding on to in relation to her father.

When Jocelyn forgave her father, a new feeling of wellbeing, personal freedom and happiness flooded into her. She has now become an active, competent leader in her retirement village and a warm, happy grandma to her grandchildren.

Isabel was 58 when she first suspected that her high-profile husband was emotionally absent even when he was physically present. He was rearranging his work schedule to be away more often, with most of his stopovers in a particular Asian city. He had to go there, he said, to get his suits made (he suddenly needed a lot of suits!). He was clearly hooked on overseas travel for the privileges that this gave him – first class travel and luxury hotels. Each time he came home was something of an anticlimax and he was already anticipating his next trip.

Isabel was finding this more and more difficult because he appeared to be bored with home life. She was beginning to dread his retirement when he would not be able to afford this five-star life and would have to come down to earth again. Any retirement activities she suggested were dismissed. Isabel confronted him. She had caught him making phone calls on his mobile to a woman in Asia. Isabel smoothed things over because she was afraid of losing her security. He was in line for a substantial superannuation package, and she had minimal independent income.

A few years later her husband's job changed dramatically because of restructuring in the organisation. He was moved 'sideways' and put in charge of the Asian region, so he needed to live there for half the year. He could have retired, but he did not want to, even though he had always said that he would retire at age 60.

In Asia he met another woman (divorced with two children). Isabel suspected that he was again hooked, but this time *he* decided to end the sham and ask her for a divorce. Fortunately, the financial settlement was amicable. She did not feel emotionally deserted *now*, because the real desertion had happened gradually over many years and she had become accepting of this. I suspect that she is still covering over her feelings but at present she is not willing to face her hurt and anger.

Some men, on reaching midlife, panic that they are missing out on something in their lives. Are their hormones failing like those of their partner's? No. But their fear is that they may be less attractive or may lose sexual performance. While this is happening, their wives are undergoing a change of shape and therefore a loss of confidence. They often feel less sexually attractive and so turn away from their partner. A man's response to this may be to look for a younger woman to bolster his ego. High-flying men who have spent a lot of time away from home living the good life come home into a more humdrum lifestyle and fear that retirement will be boring. At home the partner has had to manage the family, and her career has had to be shelved or modified. He finds her less exciting, perhaps bogged down in domesticity, even though this has been her second choice anyway. She would have liked to be a high flyer in her own right. When she has accompanied him on his overseas trips she has been an appendage. He does not spend time doing things with her but she must go to boring dinners with his boring colleagues who speak a different language. She goes off with the other wives as a tourist.

At menopause a woman may feel that she is 'old hat' or 'unwanted baggage'. She already feels less desirable, so when he leaves with a younger (sometimes exotic and foreign) woman, she is then precipitated into a real midlife crisis, which is not hormonal but emotional. She feels abandoned, useless and unwanted – past her use-by date. This is almost purely emotional turmoil and she does not need HRT for her feelings of worthlessness or panic unless there are more definite menopause symptoms occurring as well. (See 'Affairs and abandonment' in Chapter 22 for a discussion of this wounding and some practical solutions.)

Morag at the age of 46 was faced with the loss of her marriage and her house when her husband went off the rails, lost his job and their savings, and then walked out to live with someone else. She had a son to put through university and needed to stay in the same area. She was working at nights and then was made redundant. One hundred and twenty job applications later she got a job, moved to a house which needed renovating and had a big mortgage. She started work on the renovations. Then came a night when it all seemed senseless. In her nightdress, at midnight, she drove her car into the bush intending to gas herself, but she realised that if she were not found for a few days she would mess up the car and would make it smell so that her children would not be able to sell it. So she drove to a phone box and, with the only coin she had with her, rang her lawyer. It was 3 am. The lawyer asked her to come to his house and there he talked to her and offered some solutions. 'There *is* a way through', he assured her.

Many years later she looks back on that night as a turning point. She was not a victim; she kept seeking another way even when she felt worthless. Women such as Morag give me hope that there is a way through despair and hopelessness. HRT can help hot flushes and sleep disturbance but cannot fix circumstances. Courage is needed, and I see women who pick themselves up, ask for help and then rescue themselves from even the most dire circumstances. And when they do this they no longer 'long for yesterday', but they are able to get on with living 'today'.

Summary

- While HRT may help many of the symptoms of menopause, some women need to receive help with their changing emotional life.
- Women experiencing lack of confidence and self-esteem and feelings of despair and loneliness need, first and foremost, validation and support from their partner and sometimes from a trained professional.
- Some women at midlife feel like 'unwanted baggage' and this feeling is exacerbated if they are abandoned by their partner.
- Midlife can be a difficult time for men too as their youth begins to fade, and they sometimes seek refuge from this loss in the arms of a younger woman.
- A willingness to look inside at the feelings of self-doubt which inevitably arise, combined with courage, are essential for moving towards a full and happy life in older age.

6

Does menopause have to be a problem?

He is happy that thinks himself so.

Latin proverb

C an menopause be a change for the better? Midlife and menopause have had negative media exposure. They seem to be linked most often with doom and gloom and possibly physical and mental death. Midlife crisis and menopausal mayhem with associated despair and disappointment are the messages that women hear in the popular press, and hormone therapy is claimed to be positively dangerous.

Doris Lessing in the first volume of her autobiography, *Under My Skin*, says:

> The dreaded menopause did not happen: my periods ended and that was it.
>
> I did not see how I could have been more fortunate. Women with this kind of history, quite a lot of us, are sometimes made to feel guilty, as if womb troubles are the proper fate of females! I am saying this for

the benefit of young women, because all the propaganda at this time is misfortune, their lives as females presented as an obstacle course with falls along the way and a debacle at the menopause. There is something not far off: a secret society of women who have had an easy time at the menopause, and without the aid of drugs, but they hardly dare say so, for their sisters will accuse them of lying, or suggest they are letting down the side.

We can understand Doris Lessing's disquiet. Many women go through menopause gently and peacefully. The good news is hardly ever reported and the bad news gets the headlines. We do not wish to medicalise menopause and suggest that everyone needs HRT or other medical intervention. But, for some women, it *is* a time of loss and change: 'an obstacle course with falls along the way and a debacle at the menopause'. In some cases:

About 50 percent of women have little disturbance … Many women rejoice in having new freedom from periods and family responsibilities.

- The controller loses control.
- The depressed one becomes suicidal.
- Relationships deteriorate, confidence evaporates.
- There is unwanted weight and dislike of body image.
- Sex drive declines: 'I'd rather read a book or go to sleep than have sex.'
- Energy decreases: 'My get up and go has got up and gone.'

Yet there *is* life during and after menopause. About 50 percent of women have little disturbance and probably do not need to take HRT. For the other 50 percent some help is needed and appropriate assessment can assist in providing this. There is much good news (even if it goes unreported). Many women rejoice in having new freedom from periods and family responsibilities. Women may be free, at last, to do their own thing: to climb mountains or learn new skills or crafts. Some embark on postgraduate degrees. One of my patients finished her PhD last year at the age of 67. Other women leave a dead marriage and find a new love as well as a new life.

A remarkable woman called Rosemary came into my office recently for a checkup. She is 50 and is perimenopausal, but has no particular symptoms. She is serene and unflappable. She was visiting from the north-east of Queensland, which is renowned for its prolonged droughts. I asked her how she could be so content living in such a dry, harsh place. She said that in such a place you can either complain or else be grateful for the good things. Like the time it rained fish! She told me that when the land temperature rises and rises there is a big updraught created, which literally sucks up the sea and its contents. Then it literally rains fish! Who could remain unhappy at such a time!

Another of my women had to leave the desert she was in.

Sue had been married for 33 years. She had her three children when she was in her early twenties. David, her husband, was in a steady job and was totally unadventurous. He came home at the same time every night, liked the same food, and rarely could be persuaded to eat out. Sex was routine and similarly unadventurous. They visited his parents for dinner every Sunday and had the same conversations every time. Sue took a part-time job to help give her children private school education. No-one went off the rails or took drugs. All have left home and have steady partners. Two are married and one has two children. At menopause Sue had no particular symptoms but had a huge sense of loss. Life was passing her by.

Sue went to a movie about tango. She was captivated. She went and took lessons. Dave was not interested in dancing lessons, despite her invitations to him. She ran away with the dancing teacher. Dave, she says, is probably sitting in his same chair at home waiting for her to come home and cook the dinner. She can picture him, she says, reading her note and being surprised that she has gone, but sure that she will come back.

She has moved interstate. Her children applaud her move as she keeps in close touch with them via her new computer (which Dave said she would never master). She came for a routine medical check. She is fit and happy. Sex is adventurous, and she uses a small dose of estrogens in the vagina to prevent dryness.

For Sue, midlife has been about beginning again, about leaving the desert. I think for her it has also rained fish.

Marion is 55. She had her last period at the age of 51. Her periods departed quietly, 'with a whimper not a bang', she says. She occasionally feels hot but is not troubled by flushes or mood changes. She came to ask if she needed HRT for any reason. Her medical history was exemplary. The only time she was ever in hospital was to have her two children. Pregnancies and labours were normal. Her family history was also one of good health. No diabetes or strokes or breast cancer. Her father died of a heart attack aged 60 but he was a smoker and did not watch his diet. Her maternal grandmother lived to 95. Her mother is 80, plays golf and bridge and walks 5 kilometres each day.

Marion's first husband, Jim, was a workaholic who was rarely home. She brought up the children and developed her own circle of friends and interests. When Jim ran off with his secretary, Marion found a new partner whom she had known socially for years. His wife had died of cancer and their two children are grown up.

Marion and John are compatible and ideally suited. Marion is happy.
She has tried some of the natural soy products but did not feel that they
helped her in any way, as she has no particular symptoms. She is not
overweight, does not smoke and her blood pressure is normal. We
measured her cholesterol and her bone density. Both are normal, in
fact, very good. Her only problem has been vaginal dryness and some
frequency of urination. These will respond well to local (vaginal)
estrogen pessaries. She does not need HRT or prescription medicines
or even natural products.

Marion is happy. What is her secret? She grew up in a happy home with
loving parents. Though her first husband was often absent she was cared
for and found ways to create her own happiness because, she says, she
has always known that she is loved.

In Chapter 26, on forgiveness, emotional barriers to happiness will
be discussed. Be reassured, those of you who have read to this point and
may have been feeling that menopause is a pathological condition. *At
least 50 percent of all women make the menopause transition without the
need for medical or psychological help!* It is a natural transition but, like
childbirth, natural is not always normal. I remember talking to a group
of women many years ago when I first started doing menopause medicine. One woman had a frown on her face and looked puzzled as I asked
for questions at the end of my talk. She said that she felt the odd one
out in the group. She had passed through this stage of life with *no*
problems at all. What were *we* all talking about? Was *she* abnormal? I
was able to reassure her that she was perfectly normal and that many
other women have no problems. As a menopause physician, my task is
to help those who are having problems physically, mentally or emotionally. But equally my task is to assure others that there need be no
pathology or problems. It can be a trouble-free passage as Doris Lessing
claims: The 'secret society of women who have had an easy time at the
menopause' need no longer be secret.

Summary

- Menopause may bring unwanted changes in mood, weight and energy levels.
- Menopause can be a change for the better.
- It may bring freedom to do other things and to make important life changes.

7

It can't be menopause –
you're too young

It is to keep one's nerves at a strain,
To dry one's eyes and laugh at a fall,
And baffled, get up and begin again.

Robert Browning (1812–1889), 'Life in a Love'

Menopause occurring before the age of 40 is called *premature*. The usual age range for menopause is between 45 and 55. Younger women whose periods cease, for no obvious reason, before the age of 40 are usually told: 'It can't be menopause – you're too young.' They are given little reassurance or information to help them cope with this major event in their lives. Their friends are still menstruating normally and don't want to hear about it.

We are still not sure why some ovaries become resistant or why some women run out of suitable eggs. An obvious reason for young women becoming menopausal is that they have had both ovaries removed.

True surgical menopause

In this first section we will look at the worst case scenario, that of young women in their thirties who have had a true surgical menopause, i.e.

removal of both ovaries and the uterus as well. These young women go suddenly from high levels of circulating estrogens and other hormones to very low levels. They therefore suffer very acute withdrawal symptoms and are at high risk of bone-density loss.

The loss of ovaries is said to protect against breast cancer since the main source of estrogens has gone, but no young woman should be refused adequate hormone replacement on these grounds. Giving a young woman hormones to replace her loss of estrogen, in my opinion, does not alter her future risk of breast cancer since she would have produced her own hormones for the next ten years or so anyway. However, careful replacement therapy is needed. Doses that are too high produce side effects such as sore breasts, fluid retention and sometimes PMS-like mood swings. The body has been used to cyclical (fluctuating) levels, so high, steady levels may be hard to tolerate. The ovaries also produce other hormones such as progesterone, the calming hormone, and testosterone, the male hormone, which helps women to maintain libido and general body energy. These two hormones are discussed throughout the book, particularly in Chapters 8 and 21. Thus, replacement of estrogen *alone* may not restore a woman's general balance and adequate sexual functioning.

In addition to these hormonal problems, castration of a young woman will often lead to considerable psychological stress. Depression and anxiety are common reactions to this enormous psychic wound. She has been relieved of her pain and/or excessive bleeding (her most likely reason for surgery is endometriosis), but now she faces a symptomatic menopause with fertility denied and sexual functioning possibly impaired. Not every young woman facing such surgery is given a clear picture of the physical and mental outcomes.

With any woman, young or older, it is a crime against that person to remove ovaries without permission and it is reprehensible to remove ovaries without a woman's full understanding that this will render her menopausal.

Ovarian failure from chemotherapy or radiotherapy

There is another group who have early menopause because of ovarian failure induced by chemotherapy or radiotherapy (usually for a cancer of the breast or lymph glands). At least if ovaries have been removed or irradiated, the diagnosis of menopause is undeniable.

Lack of ova

Less common is ovarian failure due to a familial lack of ova (eggs). There may be a family history of mother or aunts or sisters who had early menopause.

Resistant Ovary Syndrome

Another cause of early menopause is some sort of auto-immune failure of ovarian response called Resistant Ovary Syndrome. We do not know why this happens and we have no way of assessing how many eggs there are or whether they are capable of responding to hormonal signals. Resistant Ovary Syndrome is puzzling and there is still no way of being sure whether it is temporary or permanent. *A woman's own story is very important, as most women do know if they are or are not producing their own hormones.*

There may be phases of no periods when hormones will show a menopausal pattern of high FSH and low estrogen levels. There may be the return of 'periods' for varying lengths of time, though ovulation is unpredictable – having intermittent bleeding does not necessarily mean that fertility has been restored. Measuring hormones on a regular basis is the only way to be sure of what is happening during this frustrating time.

Sometimes a woman with Resistant Ovary Syndrome does become pregnant when this is least expected, though this is rare. Younger women with this syndrome are advised to use the pill as their HRT if they do not wish to become pregnant. It is not known whether this condition represents low numbers of eggs or failure of the eggs to respond appropriately to the stimulation of the pituitary hormones, FSH and LH, as in a normal menstrual cycle. It is possibly an auto-immune problem akin to thyroid failure, where the thyroid tissue produces antibodies against itself. But whereas we can measure thyroid antibodies we cannot measure ovarian antibodies (if they even exist).

Michelle was 34 when I first met her. She had had five different operations, which bit by bit had removed her uterus and both her ovaries. She had suffered from endometriosis since her teens. She had hoped to have children but was unable to conceive. At her final operation she was told that she would be menopausal but 'a bit of estrogen for six months or so will fix this'. Within days of the operation she had almost continuous hot flushes as well as sleep disturbance, depressed mood and anxiety attacks. She was given a small dose of estrogen. It did little to relieve her symptoms.

She saw another doctor who inserted an estrogen implant. This relieved her symptoms but her breasts became very sore. Three months later, without any prior measurement of hormones, an even bigger dose implant was inserted. She now had very painful full breasts and could not bear to be touched. Sexual intercourse was painful because the vagina felt dry despite the high levels of estrogen in the rest of her body. Sexual desire had disappeared. She was not depressed now, but irritable and frustrated. She did not believe that she would ever feel normal again. She was also angry that she had not been warned about the consequences of surgically induced menopause. Her husband had been very supportive throughout her ordeals but he was becoming frustrated sexually. He thought of leaving her. He had a brief affair, but came back and talked about it to her. They went to a sexual counsellor but nothing helpful was said.

We measured her hormone levels and found estrogens over the top of the normal range. Testosterone levels were very low and most of the hormone was 'bound' i.e. not available. A month's treatment with tamoxifen, an anti-estrogen, reduced the estrogen activity in her breasts. Estrogen suppositaries in her vagina improved vaginal moisture. A testosterone implant gave her energy and sexual drive. Two months later, when her blood levels of estrogen were subsiding, a smaller implant of estrogen was tried and this did not give her undue breast tenderness. But, most important of all, proper information and careful monitoring of her blood levels, together with judicious use of lower doses of hormones, gave her mental confidence as well as physical comfort.

Michelle is now 40. She has completed a university degree and is happily teaching. Her husband agrees that menopause is not the end, and can be a new beginning.

By contrast, Lydia did not have a sudden precipitated menopause but a steady decline in ovarian function. She had been given HRT but her quality of life was poor because the doses were not carefully monitored.

Lydia was 36 when I first saw her. She had written out her gynaecological history for me and it was a tale of woe. From the age of thirteen, when she first started periods, the menstrual cycle had been a problem for her. Periods were unpredictable, bleeding was often heavy and she had pain, which interfered with school and later work attendance. Lydia needed the oral contraceptive pill to control her cycle in her teens. She ceased it to fall pregnant but her periods did not come back. Her hormone levels were low so she was given an ovarian stimulant. After she ceased this she fell pregnant naturally (and rather miraculously!). Her periods did not return after her baby was weaned. More ovarian stimulation was given. Then a spontaneous pregnancy occurred, but foetal abnormality was found on the ultrasound at 18 weeks, so a difficult termination was performed. This was emotionally as well as physically taxing.

Lydia was then referred for further fertility treatment, with success in the sixth cycle. Her periods did not come back after this pregnancy. Many different oral contraceptive pills were tried. Her hormones were at postmenopausal levels. Despite apparently adequate doses of oral hormones, her energy remained low. Every now and then she had a spontaneous surge of energy suggesting that her ovaries had switched on, but it was only for two weeks and then she would fall again in a heap.

Her hormone levels were all low when I saw her and her libido was zero. Estrogen and testosterone implants in the abdominal wall produced a huge improvement, though a skin rash may have been partly due to the testosterone, so she is now using a testosterone cream, which gives a lower level of testosterone in the blood. Lydia had begun to doubt if she would ever manage this menopausal mayhem and she often felt unheard.

This young woman's case demonstrates the difficulty in managing *intermittent* ovarian failure. Thank goodness this is not a common condition.

I must repeat that a woman's story is very important, as most women *do* know if they are producing their own hormones. There is often a strong psychological element in these cases. Lydia is a perfectionist and a high achiever, which also means that she is often disappointed and frustrated. I suspect that this type of personality has some effect on the hormonal pattern though it does not usually cause early menopause. I have noted in my practice that such women are more likely to suffer from PMS or endometriosis.

Frustration is understandable, as the young woman is never quite sure what is happening. It must therefore be galling to know that *some* women have so little problem with their menstrual cycle and fall pregnant with consummate ease!

Doris Lessing was one of these and she says in her book, *Under My Skin*:

My gynaecological history would be appropriate for that fabled peasant woman who has never had anything wrong with her. I had my first period when I was fourteen. My periods lasted two or three days and were never excessive. They were sometimes mildly painful. As for premenstrual tension, no-one had ever heard of it.

I gave birth three times and was never torn, stitched, forcepped, or caesared. I have never suffered from thrush or herpes. My periods ceased in my early forties, as is common for women who smoke.

She then talks about how easy menopause was for her:

Here is the point, and if I am labouring it, then it is because I believe it to be important: when I, my generation, looked forward to our lives as females, we were not full of fear and foreboding. We felt confident, we felt in control. We were not bombarded with bleak information from television, radio, newspapers, and women's magazines.

What Lessing says is probably true to an extent but, on the other hand, a lot of women of her generation would have lacked awareness, suffered in silence and sought no help, or alternatively there would not have been much that could have been done to help them.

In this book we try to present both sides of the picture, to assure women that they can, indeed, sail through their reproductive lives with few or no problems. But I do not believe that appropriate information causes women to fear and thus perform badly. This is really a case where 'a *little* knowledge is a dangerous thing', especially if the information is slanted and only the negative receives attention. I hope that this book dispels some myths and puts truth in their place, especially for younger women.

It would be useful, here, to refer to the diagrams in Chapter 1, which explain women's hormonal fluctuations. In these it appeared that hormones seemed to be the main cause of the problems. But a woman's personality also reacts with her hormones and we all have to take responsibility for our own attitudes. Michelle needed hormone replacement and she also had to come to terms with her own frustrations. Lydia was conducting a sort of war with her hormones. She only found peace when she gave up the fight. It seems to be a matter, as quoted earlier in the chapter, of 'baffled, get up and begin again'. To do this requires good information and reassurance.

Summary

- Premature menopause occurs with the removal of both ovaries and the uterus, and may also be brought on by ovarian failure.
- Ovarian failure may be induced by chemotherapy or radiotherapy, a familial lack of ova or Resistant Ovary Syndrome.
- Careful hormone replacement therapy, based on individual assessment, is necessary for the successful management of young menopausal women.
- Hormones appear to be the main cause of problems in these young women, although psychological factors probably do play a part.

8

War and peace –
menstrual mayhem and PMS

There has never been a war yet which, if the facts had been presented before
ordinary folk, could not have been prevented.

Ernest Bevin (1881–1951), British Labour leader and statesman

Some women struggle all their reproductive lives with their hormones. It is literally a bloody war and the hormones win most of the rounds. Peace is what we all hope for, but this can only come about by prevention of war. This chapter attempts to give younger premenopausal women information about why the hormonal warfare occurs. Only then can prevention begin.

Women were never meant to have menstruation except in the intervals between having babies and breastfeeding. We are, these days, trying to subvert our biological destiny. But being continuously reproductive, i.e. being either pregnant or breastfeeding from the age of 16 to the age of 40, has one great advantage: it saves a lot of menstrual mayhem. The 'primitive' women of New Guinea who begin their reproductive careers at age 16, when their periods first start, are either pregnant or breastfeeding most of the time thereafter, having very few periods in their whole reproductive lifetime. We 'civilised' women start periods at an average age of 12 and go on with periods with very little break (two or three pregnancies only) until we arrive at menopause at the average age of 52. Nearly 40 years of unused cycles! It is likely that 'what you don't use you lose' and the high rate of hysterectomy bears this out. Few women these days want to be pregnant most of their reproductive lives, as their great-grandmothers probably were, so there has to be another way to manage menstrual cycles that start to disrupt normal life.

One of the crippling menstrual disorders of our modern society is premenstrual syndrome (PMS), also called premenstrual tension (PMT). In some instances, emotional or psychological symptoms predominate and the term Premenstrual Dysphoric Disorder (PMDD) is used. PMS is under-researched, so exact definitions, classifications and treatments are still being debated. But we do know that many women suffer from it. Families and friends also suffer and the workplace may also be disrupted by this disorder of modern society. Some women seek help fearing/hoping that it is early menopause. I must say that the menopause is easier to bear than the debilitating effects of PMS and I tell women this, because some feel that if PMS is so unbearable maybe menopause will be even worse. At least with menopause we can measure hormones and make a diagnosis, and HRT usually gives relief.

So what is this disorder called PMS that affects about 25 percent of women by the age of 35? You will note that I call it a disorder, not a disease. Disorder implies that a natural process is out of order. Disease usually indicates that there is an outside agency at work transmitted by bacteria or viruses (e.g. glandular fever, pelvic infection etc.).

PMS seems to be an abnormal response to hormones and it is strictly cyclical, being related to the second half of the cycle, reaching a peak before menstruation and subsiding as bleeding begins. There are physical symptoms such as fluid retention, abdominal bloating and sugar cravings, but it is the emotional/mental symptoms that are the most disturbing and disruptive elements. Abrupt mood swings, anger, irritability, clumsiness and loss of self-esteem lead to abnormal, and at times bizarre, behaviour. Women themselves recognise that they are some of the time Mr Hyde, but increasingly Dr Jekyll. The poet, Alexander Pope, must have had personal experience of women's vagaries when he said, 'Woman's at best a contradiction still.'

PMS is certainly a situation where women ask the question, 'Is it me or my hormones?' It is both. Women who are perfectionists are more likely to suffer the emotional symptoms. Women who are estrogen sensitive (who in pregnancy had severe nausea or marked fluid retention) are more likely to have the physical symptoms. One theory that has been around for 50 years or so is that an estrogen/progesterone imbalance, with a preponderance of estrogen, is the major cause. Dr Katherina Dalton and Wendy Hilton and, more recently, Dr John Lee have written extensively about this. They each have many followers, but I do not believe that there is one single hormone deficiency that is a cause for this variegated and variable disorder. Rather it is an interaction between the woman and her hormones.

Dr Dalton, an English medical practitioner who first came to fame in the 1950s, believed strongly that lack of progesterone in the second half of the menstrual cycle could cause women to behave in uncharacteristic ways. She was able to get some women's court sentences reduced after they had committed crimes such as shoplifting, using the hormonal changes as the reason for their behaviour. Dr Lee, an American medical practitioner, wrote a small monograph about progesterone some ten years ago, which was initially circulated privately. He has subsequently written several books for a general audience in which he claims that 'estrogen dominance' (which implies relative progesterone lack) is responsible for most premenopausal symptoms and especially PMS. He also asserts in these books that progesterone deficiency is the main cause of menopausal symptoms and he strongly advocates the use of this hormone as HRT. Unfortunately, many products marketed as yam creams,

> As women approach the age of 37 ... ovulation starts to falter, so progesterone production may be less than it was ... it is around this age that major PMS occurs.

which claim to contain progesterone and thus supply its lack in the body, do not contain progesterone itself but its precursor, diosgenin, which is not active in the human body.

Some gynaecologists and endocrinologists still believe that the *presence* rather than the absence of progesterone is the cause of PMS symptoms because the symptoms occur in the second half of the cycle, the luteal phase, when progesterone normally kicks in after ovulation occurs. But if the presence of the progesterone in the second half of the cycle is the cause rather than *lack* of progesterone, why do not more young women in their teens and twenties have *major* PMS? They certainly have recognisable mood changes and breast soreness, but it is not usually a major problem. It is interesting to note that they are in the peak reproductive phase when ovulation is present in most cycles.

As women approach the age of 37, however, ovulation starts to falter, so progesterone production may be less than it was. And it is around this age that major PMS occurs.

Measuring hormone levels can be very confusing. During the menstrual cycle there is so much variation from day to day in a normal cycle that one measurement in a cycle is hard to interpret. As women move into their late thirties, ovulation may occur only haphazardly, causing progesterone levels to be low. This is linked, I believe, with the hormonal mayhem that we call PMS. It also causes infertility.

A group of 20 women was followed for 20 years, from age 35 to 55, by one of the major Australian researchers, Professor Jim Brown. Hormone levels in the urine were measured weekly and symptoms recorded. It was clear that even though periods *seemed* to be normal, hormone levels were varying from day to day and cycle to cycle. The changes were subtle and there was often relative progesterone deficiency, with the symptoms that we call PMS being more likely in those cycles of *relative* progesterone deficiency.

A woman's own story must also be heard. What she is experiencing in her life cannot be denied. The physical symptoms are often obvious, but the emotional and psychological symptoms are harder to assess.

Melissa is aged 38. She is desperate. For 10 to 12 days premenstrually she changes into a screaming banshee. Crockery is thrown. Her children avoid her and her husband comes home late and tries to sneak into the house. Her periods seem fairly regular and normal, though sometimes bleeding is heavier. She has successfully combined career and motherhood. She had her children when she was in her mid-thirties. After each child she had postnatal depression, though this was not recognised at the time. She is a solicitor, working in an all-male practice. She feels clumsy in her premenstrual phase and sometimes makes mistakes. She had her tubes tied after her last child. She was on the Pill in her twenties and had no side effects. She is a perfectionist. Her PMS alarms and distresses her because she feels unable to control the savage moods. She has always been a high achiever and a fierce competitor.

Melissa did not really want to go back on the Pill. She had been told that it is not suitable for women over 35. That is why she had her tubes tied. I persuaded her to use it again. The Pill suppresses her own cycle and gives her a constant steady level of hormones. Within three months she settled and found it hard to believe that she had been such a shrew. How long can she take the Pill? There is no definite time limit, but most women try without it after a year or so. Some seem to settle as they go into their forties; some don't. A few women need to stay on the pill right up to menopause. Their partners and children are grateful.

Jane is 41. Like Melissa, she is a professional woman. She postponed pregnancy so that she could do a postgraduate degree and now has a two-year-old daughter. Her parents and her husband's parents live in another state, so there are no grandparents available to offer assistance with her daughter. She and John, her husband, have pursued separate successful careers. They have a large house and two cars, and have been used to having holidays abroad each year. They employ a babysitter to look after their daughter. Jane comes home rather late, cooks dinner and puts the baby to bed. By the time John comes home she is too tired to talk to him, or if she talks she screams. She is too tired and fraught to have sex. He finds this difficult, so refuses to talk to her. Her periods are heavier than they used to be. Premenstrually her breasts are very sore. But it is the mental symptoms that disturb her most. Her moods swing wildly. She has very little time for herself and resents this. The baby that she so desired seems to have irretrievably altered her whole life. She does very little exercise. She binge eats and drinks a lot of coffee.

The initial approach here was for Jane to alter her lifestyle – to cut down on caffeine and alcohol intake, particularly in the last half of her cycle. She now goes to a gym twice a week and has also cut down her working hours. John is coming home from work earlier as well. They have made Sunday a rest day. Jane has been using a progesterone cream and this seems to have helped her moods, but the lifestyle changes must be credited with the major part of her improvement. *Hormones cannot compete with a busy driven woman!*

Many other treatments have been suggested for the management of PMS. These include evening primrose oil (this helps breast soreness as it has an action similar to that of aspirin), vitamin B6, magnesium, calcium, and a variety of herbs, including black cohosh, ginseng and vitex agnus castus, but apart from the last-named, few of these have been subjected to rigorous scientific examination.

In the last few years the other type of PMS has been recognised which, as mentioned above, we call Premenstrual Dysphoric Disorder (PMDD). This condition has a preponderance of emotional swings rather than physical symptoms, such as breast soreness, and for some women may occupy more than just a week or two premenstrually. The classic symptoms are anxiety, irritability and mood swings, with resulting loss of self-esteem. It is not surprising that all these things lead to a feeling of guilt and can cause quite severe family disruption. For PMDD, mood-altering drugs such as SSRIs (selective serotonin uptake inhibitors) may be needed to treat the hormone changes occurring in the hypothalamus. Psychotherapy is also useful for exploring patterns of behaviour. I have noted in my own practice that sexual abuse in childhood and teenage years carries a high risk of menstrual dysfunction and mood disorder in later life.

Mary-Anne, aged 39, came to see me because of 'bad PMT for three weeks per month'. She had been given HRT in an attempt to 'straighten out' her aberrant hormones. This made her much worse, as she had now developed sore breasts and bloating, which had not been a problem with her own hormones. Hormone measurement showed low estrogen levels on only one occasion, so this was not menopause. I took her off the HRT, rechecked her hormone levels three times in her next cycle and found that she had fairly normal highs and lows, and was certainly not menopausal. I discussed the use of fluoxetine with her, but she was reluctant, at first, to try this as she felt it was an antidepressant and therefore unacceptable. Next month she came back to see me and decided to take this medication. Prozac is one trade name for fluoxetine. It was developed initially as an antidepressant and then found to have other mood-altering effects. It is one of many drugs which selectively alter serotonin levels in the brain.

Three months later Mary-Anne came back and thanked me for helping to get her life back. The family could not believe the difference, nor could she.

There is still, in developed countries, a great antagonism to the use of antidepressants or any mood-altering medications because of the fear that 'I may get addicted' and 'I can't be shown to have any mental weakness – what will my family think, what will my friends say?' There is still this stigma attached to any form of perceived 'mental' illness. Physical conditions can be coped with and talked about, but mental problems must be secret as they are seen to be shameful.

It is this conspiracy of silence that has hampered the appropriate treatment of women's breakdowns occurring at times of hormonal deprivation or change, such as postnatal depression, PMDD and menopause. As mentioned earlier in this chapter, we are exposed, nowadays, to hormonal shifts and surges that nature did not intend us to have. We really should be pregnant or breastfeeding all our reproductive lives. Menstrual periods with their hormonal upsets are actually not what nature intended, so treatment is not an admission of failure on our part, but rather a recognition of the fact that hormonal swings can cause problems. *Understanding and reassurance are vital ingredients in the successful management of the distressing and puzzling problems, PMS and PMDD, which afflict at least 5 percent of women to a severe degree and probably 40 percent to a lesser degree.*

PMS is not menopause but a premenopausal change in hormone balance, usually starting in the mid-thirties and lasting for five to ten years. I have heard it described as 'the change before the change'. One of my patients called it 'the scourge of the middle ages'. In some ways it is worse than menopause because measuring hormone levels does not always give a clue to what is happening. It needs repeated measurements over many cycles and that is not always practicable.

So, 'Is it me or my hormones?' I think it is both. A certain kind of woman is more likely to get PMS or PMDD. She is usually a perfectionist; she is often trying to be model mother, wife and career woman. She may have grown up with some messages from her parents that make her try to go beyond her own limits. She may have been prey to sexual abuse. So can war give way to peace? I believe that it can and that the menstrual and psychic mayhem can be managed through lifestyle changes and appropriate medication. Many women, as well as men, will be relieved to hear this.

Summary

- Biologically, women are not meant to menstruate almost continually throughout their lives; however, this is neither practicable nor necessary in today's world.
- This is thought to be a major reason for the menstrual disorders of modern society, premenstrual stress (PMS) and Premenstrual Dysphoric Disorder (PMDD).
- Estrogen/progesterone imbalance has been cited as a cause of PMS, but there are those who believe that it is caused by a hormonal/psychological interaction.
- PMS is an abnormal response to hormones and is strictly cyclical, with both physical symptoms and emotional symptoms.
- PMS can respond positively to lifestyle changes, the Pill and/or fluoxetine (Prozac).
- The symptoms of PMDD are predominantly emotional and may respond better to fluoxetine and/or psychotherapy.
- It is believed that women who are perfectionists are more likely to suffer from the emotional symptoms, and women who are estrogen sensitive are more prone to the physical symptoms.

9

Oops! I forgot to have kids!

I once told a magazine writer that I intended to be childless all my life because I didn't want to trip over any little feet on my way to the top.

Anna Quindlen, *One True Thing*

It is the cause of much distress for those women who have knowingly postponed childbearing in favour of other things, such as their careers, which appeared to be more important or fulfilling, to find that they are experiencing perimenopause and their fertility is markedly reduced. If a woman does not heed her biological clock, it keeps on ticking, and then just when she is at last ready to have a baby, it appears that she is no longer fertile. Her dream is shattered.

Women need to be reminded that they are built to have babies in their early twenties when reproductive capacity is at its peak.

We know that some of our grandmothers kept on having babies into their forties. But they had these babies at the end of the reproductive line, not at the beginning. In this way they had also provided other children who could help mother these younger children while they were going through menopause. And their reproductive function was like a well-oiled machine which worked, as it should, without missing a beat. These were the women who longed for menopause to escape from unavoidable childbearing!

What has happened? What has gone wrong? Women in their late thirties now appear to be less fertile than their grandmothers at that age.

Theories abound about it being due to external pollutants, petrochemicals in the atmosphere, estrogens in our food, the oral contraceptive pill, etc., etc. But in most cases it is simply that the biological clock has passed midday and the sun is moving towards setting. It is the internal environment rather than the external that is at fault. The decision to delay pregnancy has mostly been a flawed one. Some women have hoped that scientific solutions will be found, like those reported in *Time Magazine* of 27 October 1997: 'Eggs on the rocks: a new procedure may offer women the chance to freeze their ova – and stop their biological clock.'

A psychosomatic component may well accompany the biological factor. I have noticed during my career of 40 years as an obstetrician and gynaecologist that the chance of getting pregnant seems to be inversely related to the desire to become pregnant or to avoid pregnancy. Not many pregnancies are truly planned. Most just happen. If it is an unlikely time to get pregnant, then it will happen; if strenuous efforts are being made to avoid it, it still may happen. Of course, some couples have successfully planned pregnancies and I am *not* saying that it was just luck – and it may well have been good management – but I have observed that when a couple desperately, even frantically, tries for pregnancy, then the very wanting and straining sometimes works against it.

So, if nature calls, it is best to take heed and not postpone pregnancy until chances are too slim. This is the major message in this chapter.

Award-winning journalist and best-selling author Anna Quindlen was in her twenties when she wrote a features column called 'About New York'. She was the first woman and the youngest person to do that column and it was at this time that she told a magazine writer that she intended to be childless all her life 'because I don't want to trip over little feet on the way to the top'. But soon she decided to take a less spectacular path and have children. In fact, she later became the only female opinion columnist for the *New York Times*, perhaps the best and

most desirable position in journalism. She wrote on the issues of the day
– abortion, health care, gay rights etc. – and by this time she had three
children under twelve. She won the Pulitzer Prize in 1992. It was then
that she started to write novels, the first being *One True Thing*. Coming
from a time in her life when she had been prepared to put her career
above having children, she now decided to put children before her
career. She gave up her day job on the *New York Times* to become a fiction writer. Someone asked her if fiction writing was satisfying enough
for her to give up a very visible job for one that is nearly invisible. She
was also accused of being afraid of success! Some said that her resignation proved that women can't have their cake and eat it too.

I think Quindlen's story shows that women *can* have it all, but
choices still have to be made. It is unfortunately true that it is possible
to miss the boat as far as having children is concerned if pregnancy is
delayed too long, as we can see in the following story.

Tracey is aged 39. She has never married, though she has had one
long-term relationship and several other 'flings' to use her term. Her
biological clock is ticking so loudly now that it is deafening her. She is
desperately searching for a man to father her child. Her present partner
is only part time and she does not feel that she wants to marry him or
have his baby. She has thought of going to a clinic and asking for
artificial insemination and then 'going it alone'. She is concerned
because her periods are very irregular and the blood loss is much less
than it used to be. Recently she went for five months without a period
and had some hot flushes. She feels mildly depressed and tired. She is
a teacher who loves her job but is often short-tempered with the
children. She is constantly reminded of her own missing motherhood.

Tracey did not at first volunteer the information that she has had
three terminations of pregnancy! The first was when she was engaged at
eighteen, but she did not then feel ready for a pregnancy. The second
was after one of her flings. She had parted from this man; in fact, he

had disappeared and she felt abandoned. The third pregnancy was to her present partner. She did not feel committed to him and he was very sure that he did not want a baby. So the pregnancy was not convenient. That was three years ago.

I asked her if she had felt any remorse over the terminations. She said that she had not felt in any way ready to go on with any of the pregnancies. She did not seek counselling. On each occasion she went in and had a termination. No regrets.

Now, suddenly, she is flooded with desire to have a child. She feels angry that she may miss out. She came demanding an answer and a solution. Her own doctor had checked her hormone levels and found them to be consistent with menopause. She had told her bluntly that she had absolutely no chance of pregnancy. I rechecked her hormones, as she had had a light bleed three weeks before I saw her. Her estrogens were low but not in the menopausal range and her FSH was not above 20. This meant that she was not absolutely menopausal. She may have a few more periods but it is unlikely that she is ovulating and pregnancy is extremely unlikely.

Maybe not for Tracey, but sometimes surprises (miracles?) do happen, as we shall see below.

Anna at the age of 37 had three ectopic pregnancies within eight months. She asked herself after this: 'Do I have to be a mother?' and her inner self answered, 'Stuff this! You haven't seen the sun come up over the Himalayas either!' But she later started on a fertility program (as a single prospective mother). At this time she met James who had two older children and he offered to be a sperm donor for her. She did not initially agree but started to go out with him socially. Three months later in Israel, at the age of 43, she fell pregnant naturally and married James, and had the baby which had seemed so unlikely.

My medical partner, Dr Anne Jequier, is an international expert in male hormones and fertility (andrology) as well as female infertility. She is the head of a fertility clinic. She sees many women who have postponed pregnancy and are now desperate. Hormone monitoring shows that even if these women are still having menstrual cycles, the cycles are not ovulatory. Usually the FSH levels are close to the upper border of normality so this means that trying to stimulate ovulation is unlikely to be effective.

Dr Jequier explains the problem as follows:

There is no doubt that problems of infertility begin in earnest when a woman is in her mid-thirties. This becomes very significant at age 37 when fertility rapidly falls. Between the ages of 38 and 40, the pregnancy rate of almost any treatment halves, while between the ages of 40 and 42 the pregnancy rate following treatment halves again. At 43 years of age the pregnancy rate following almost any treatment, but certainly IVF, is less than 5 percent. It is likely by 44 years to be as little as 1 percent.

A major factor in determining pregnancy rate is a past pregnancy, suggesting that only those who have previously achieved a pregnancy are likely to conceive when this age is reached.

An important indicator of success of any form of treatment, but particularly IVF, can be seen in the FSH level measured on day two or day three. FSH stands for Follicle Stimulating Hormone, which is produced by the pituitary. It rises and falls during the menstrual cycle and it stimulates the follicle(s) in the ovary to secrete estrogen in preparation for ovulation. When there are no more follicles available, the FSH rises well above 20, periods cease or tail off and this is menopause. A raised level on either day two or three of the cycle (and *only* on these two days of the cycle) results in a poor pregnancy rate. Indeed, experts have demonstrated that if the day two level of FSH exceeds 15 units per litre then an IVF pregnancy has never been achieved.

Levels of FSH between 10 and 15 units are commonly seen in unstimulated women of 38 years or more and even these indicate a poor prognosis for pregnancy.

When an older woman attempts to achieve a pregnancy using IVF, a number of different problems may arise. In women of 38 or more there is a reduction in the number of eggs obtained after stimulation as well as a reduction in egg quality. Then the percentage of eggs that are fertilised is reduced, so there are fewer embryos than in the younger women undergoing IVF, and those embryos may also be of poorer quality (with a higher rate of abnormality). There may be failure to respond to gonadotrophin therapy (FSH injections etc.) for two main reasons.

Firstly, the response to stimulation may be poor and huge doses of gonadotrophin are needed to generate only one or two mature eggs. (Younger women may produce a dozen eggs.)

Secondly, the gonadotrophin therapy may actually *reduce* estrogen levels. (It normally increases them markedly.) It would appear that the FSH treatment acts by down-regulating the ovaries in much the same way as that seen in young women with Resistant Ovary Syndrome. This response may even be seen among women with apparently normal cycles who appear to be ovulating spontaneously. I have never seen a pregnancy in a woman with this type of response.

What measures can be taken by a younger woman to safeguard her fertility into the fourth decade? *What this woman must remember is that there is no technique that will guarantee fertility at any time of life, but there are techniques that can be used that will give a better prognosis for pregnancy than that normally seen at 40 years of age.*

The first of these options is that egg production is stimulated and eggs collected in exactly the same way as that used in IVF. These eggs can now be fertilised to become embryos that can then be cryopreserved ('put on ice').

In some Western countries, embryos have a limited 'shelf life', i.e. they cannot be kept frozen for longer than a prescribed time. In most states of Australia, for example, this is 5 years, so this would hardly be practicable in a woman who did not wish to have children until she was 45 years of age (i.e. if she produces her embryos in her twenties or thirties and then delays pregnancy until her forties). She would also, of course, have to be in a stable relationship with the same partner or such embryos may not at a later date be acceptable to her.

The second option is that we cryopreserve unfertilised eggs ('eggs on the rocks'). This achieves a poorer pregnancy rate than that achieved with frozen embryos.

Unfertilised eggs take poorly to freezing; their fragile membranes and, worse, their chromosomes may be damaged. This is in marked contrast to sperms which can readily be frozen and remain viable for years. However, it has recently been demonstrated that freezing of more immature eggs (eggs that are at an early stage of division) and their subsequent maturation and fertilisation in vitro (outside the body, in a test tube) may give rise to a better pregnancy rate than that achieved to date.

The third option is the use of cryopreserved ovarian tissue and the very immature follicles contained within it. It has now been shown that this tissue can be transplanted following storage, but no pregnancy has yet been achieved from such transplants. Likewise, we are still a long way from achieving maturation of these primordial follicles in vitro (in the test tube). This technique has been suggested for young women who lose ovarian function due to surgical removal of ovaries, or due to radiotherapy or chemotherapy for various kinds of cancer. Primordial follicles are the egg cells in the state that they are in while still in the ovary, before they have been stimulated by the pituitary-stimulating hormones, FSH and LH. They are potential eggs.

The last, and perhaps the least acceptable, option is to use eggs that have been donated by a younger woman. Such eggs can then be fertilised using the husband's sperm and are then transferred to the woman's uterus after suitable hormonal preparation of that womb. This is the technique which is used in the clinic in Rome where women in their sixties have achieved pregnancies.

Another similar option is to use donated embryos that have been discarded by women who have undergone IVF and have achieved the family number they wanted, so have embryos to spare. It must be remembered that in some states of Australia *one is not allowed to use IVF to treat infertility that is the result of age alone.* Thus it is important that such legislative prohibitions be taken into account.

Above all, it must be remembered that whatever technique is preferred, fertility cannot be guaranteed, especially later in life, and that the best option is to undertake pregnancy at an earlier age when the risks of infertility, the risks of pregnancy itself and the risks of congenital abnormality are so much lower.

Such schemes as outlined above for what we could call a 'maternity insurance' come at a price. Delaying childbearing until the forties increases some obstetric risks such as high blood pressure, and the older mother has then to raise the child when she is going through her menopause.

From Anne's exposition above, it is clear that these days there are more women who are losing their fertility at an earlier age. As mentioned earlier in the chapter, we are not sure why this is – most of the theories have been extrapolated from animal populations. We cannot really attribute it to external agents. Perhaps we should be looking instead at the internal agents such as undue stress. Women these days are not entirely content with the motherhood role only, but want a career as well. There is conflict in this, which may well adversely affect reproductive function. But the reality is that women should be encouraged to obey the dictates of nature and have their babies when their fertility is still high, which is the conclusion reached by Dr Jequier from her clinical experience.

My advice to Tracey in the earlier story was that, although a spontaneous pregnancy was not *completely* out of the question, it was extremely unlikely. Stimulation of ovulation was not likely to be successful either, as the problem seemed to be that her ova were either now very few or were not responding to stimulation from her pituitary gland. She did seem to be heading for a premature menopause. Of course, fertility clinics can provide other options such as egg donation. But whose sperm does she use? Is this really warranted just because a woman is desperate? There are some ethical questions here that are, as yet, unanswered. Any way we look at this, it is too late for Tracey to store eggs or embryos as mentioned above. Even more important than the practicalities and possibilities is the fact that Tracey needs to look at her *reaction* to her predicament. She needs to deal with her anger and disappointment – otherwise she may be heading for a psychological breakdown.

Summary

- Women who delay pregnancy until well into their thirties often have difficulty conceiving as the fertility rate declines rapidly from around 37 years of age.
- Women need to be aware that their reproductive capacity is at its peak in their early twenties.
- Some believe that the additional stress women experience today from high-powered careers, for example, may be contributing to loss of fertility at an earlier age.
- Women can have both career and children, but a choice needs to be made sufficiently early for them to conceive. If not, women may have to deal with feelings of anger, disappointment and grief.

Part 2

Symptoms and treatment of menopause

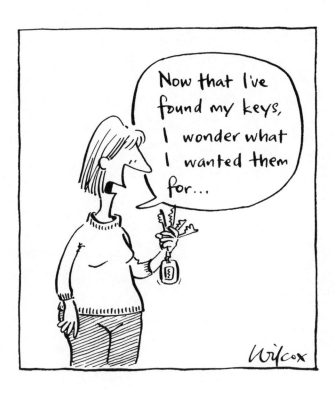

10

Swings and roundabouts –
getting the balance right with treatment

What I dream of is an art of balance, of purity and serenity devoid of troubling or depressing subject matter ... a soothing, calming influence on the mind, rather like a good armchair which provides relaxation from physical fatigue.

Henri Matisse (1869–1954)

In midlife some women seem to lose balance and serenity. Loss of balance may be physical, as one of the symptoms of menopausal hormone deficiency is dizziness. At this time also, blood pressure may be creeping up and causing light-headedness or dizziness. Or it may be emotional, as moods swing widely and do not seem to settle in the middle where they should be: that point where there is control, calmness and coping. How we all long for this! Menopause therapists, whether they give HRT or herbs, are keen to get the balance right. Too much may give side effects; too little will not relieve symptoms.

A report on the 1999 Australasian Menopause Society Congress was called 'Getting the Balance Right'. It is encouraging to know that medical experts recognise that balance is important and that therapy needs to be individualised. It is not enough for a doctor to take a packet of HRT out of his drawer and ask his patient to use it without that doctor thinking carefully about the woman's personal needs and the possible side effects. The product information contained within this packet is often alarming, since it has to list everything that has ever happened to anyone who has taken this medication, without any real critical analysis as to whether this is really of any relevance to the majority of users. To add to this problem, much of the small print data relates to the *synthetic* hormones of the oral contraceptive pill. The pharmaceutical companies feel that they must cover every eventuality. Thus not all of their information applies directly to HRT because HRT uses smaller doses of either estradiol or estrone. These are hormones produced in a laboratory but are of the same basic structure as our natural hormones. The small print on the medication packet inserts needs explanation from the doctor who prescribes it, as it may alarm the patient who is not given a proper assessment of benefits as well as risks. Again, we need to stress, treatment needs to be individualised.

So how do we get the balance right?

Dawn came to see me recently. She is aged 45. She had a hysterectomy a year ago. One ovary was removed because of cysts. One ovary remains. This ovary should presumably function for the term of its natural life (until age 45 to 50). But very soon after the operation, Dawn began to have hot flushes and undue tiredness. Her doctor assumed that these symptoms were due to menopause and put in an estrogen implant. Within a week the hot flushes were replaced by extreme breast soreness and swelling. She became cranky and irritable. Her doctor prescribed evening primrose oil and gave her some progestogen tablets. The breast pain gradually subsided. After four months she felt more comfortable but her breasts were still enlarged and tender. She had a long history of 'busy' breasts, with premenstrual swelling and pain. She had had many breast cysts drained. Her mother had a mastectomy for breast cancer at age 65 but is now 75 and well. There is no other family history of breast cancer.

The hot flushes returned and Dawn felt mildly depressed. Another doctor persuaded her to try a serial-type oral HRT, but once again her breasts responded dramatically to this medication as the dose of estrogen was still high. I saw her at this stage.

Dawn had seen a naturopath but the prescribed herbals were not helping her symptoms. Her sex life was virtually nonexistent due to a combination of discomforts. She could not bear her husband to touch her breasts or hug her, she felt tired and nonreactive sexually, and her vagina was dry and uncomfortable. She asked for help with the hot flushes but adamantly (and wisely) refused HRT. I agreed with her that hormones in normal doses were not a good idea. I gave her tamoxifen, an anti-estrogen, which is used for breast cancers which are estrogen related. It is also on long-term trial as an estrogen antagonist in women with possible increased risk of breast cancer, such as a significant family history. I warned her that this would not help and may even aggravate the hot flushes, but she thought this was a small price to pay for relief of the breast pain. Within weeks her breasts had shrunk and become comfortable. I gave her local estrogen pessaries to relieve the vaginal dryness and this was also very effective. Her husband was able to get close and even hug her. Sex was possible, though she still felt that her libido was lacking.

We checked her hormone levels every few weeks and found that she was having estrogen swings, so not all the breast activity was due to the HRT but to the surging of her own hormones produced by the remaining ovary. She noted that her hot flushes were waxing and waning, so it was most likely that just when she had that first big dose of estrogen as an implant she had her own surge. It is no wonder that her levels of estrogen went right over the top and that her breasts were grossly overstimulated. This also accounted for her emotional irritability. A few months later, when the hot flushes came back, she was able to tolerate estrogen in the smallest dose patch and at this stage her hormone levels were truly menopausal, so HRT could be given without side effects.

It is important to achieve a balance for every individual because breasts are more responsive in some women than others and hormone levels may still be coming and going. To arrive at a balance is to put hot flushes on one side of the scale and breast soreness and overactivity on the other. In practice, this means giving doses that will relieve the flushes without creating undue breast activity. We doctors need to 'titrate' the dose against the effects as we were taught in pharmacy. (I graduated in medicine in a bygone era when we actually made up our own medicines.)

Breast soreness does not increase the risk of getting breast cancer, but estrogens do make sensitive breast cells grow and divide ...

In Dawn's case there was another question to answer. Did the breast overactivity induced by estrogen pose any increased risk of breast cancer? Many women have heard that this is so. Dawn was already rather anxious because of her mother's history of breast cancer. We can reassure women that breast soreness does not increase the risk of getting breast cancer, but estrogens do make sensitive breast cells grow and divide, as we have mentioned in earlier chapters, so any existing cancer that is estrogen sensitive may grow more rapidly when exposed to estrogen therapy.

Very active breasts also make mammography screening difficult, as the breast tissue is very dense, and fine detail may be obscured. It is worth saying, at this point, that breast ultrasound is not a replacement for mammography. It is used in women with dense breasts, or obvious cysts, to define the cysts and perhaps aid in aspiration of them. Ultrasound will not show up the fine patterns of calcification, which are diagnostic of very early cancer before any mass is palpable. Mammography and ultrasound are complementary not alternative modes of diagnosis.

The take-home message is: try to avoid over-stimulating the breasts with hormones.

Since we began writing this book another HRT has come on the market in Australia called tibolone (trade name Livial), which was mentioned in Chapter 4. This has been available in the UK for ten years and is marketed as 'The HRT that you take when you do not want to take estrogen'. It is a steroid molecule that has some of the actions of the main sex hormones (i.e. estrogen, progesterone and testosterone) but it is none of these. Clinical evidence suggests that it relieves many menopause symptoms without causing breast soreness, as HRT does, and without stimulating the breasts or the lining of the uterus. This makes it ideal. Many specialists believe that it improves bone density, reduces flushes and sweats and vaginal dryness, and improves libido. It is not used before menopause or during the menopause transition when bleeding is still likely. It would seem to be ideal for women who have breasts that over-respond to estrogens. Probably it could be used, also, for women who have had breast cancer and are now suffering severe symptoms of menopause and have been told not to take estrogens. A specific study to show that it is safe for these women had not been done when it was first released but is now in progress.

Jessie was sent to me because she had osteoporosis of her spine. This was picked up on bone-density measurement, which was done because her mother had had osteoporosis and had fractured her hip. Jessie was now 70. She had had an easy menopause and did not need HRT. She has always exercised moderately and has a good diet, which is high in calcium. Her doctor started her on HRT at a moderately high dose of both estrogen and progestogen. She developed acutely sore breasts and abdominal bloating. In fact she felt wretched! This dose of HRT is the one used in the osteoporosis trials. It has been shown to prevent further bone-density loss and even increase it slowly over time, so many physicians assume that this dose must be used to treat osteoporosis and that any lesser dose may not be adequate. But Jessie's body got a shock! It had been used to very low levels of estrogen for 20 years so it responded angrily. Jessie stopped taking the hormones saying that she would risk a fracture rather than become 'a Dolly Parton'!

We X-rayed her upper (thoracic) spine – that is, the spine in her chest. Spinal bone density can only be measured on the lower part of the spine, the lumbar, as the ribs are included in the picture and confuse it if we try to measure the vertebrae in the chest part of the spine. Yet the thoracic vertebrae are the very ones we need to know about because this is where fracture often occurs, causing the deformity that we call the 'dowager's hump'.

Jessie had cracks already appearing in these vertebrae. The front end of a vertebra is the weakest part. The back end has the spinal processes for support, which make it stronger. Thus she had the earliest evidence of fracture, though it was not yet causing symptoms. Backache is felt when the fracture starts to cause the 'dowager's hump'. This deformity is irreversible. It should be prevented by treating osteoporosis before a fracture has occurred.

We started Jessie on a non-hormonal medication, alendronate (trade name, Fosamax), which not only stops bone loss, but also increases bone density. The alternative, if we could have persuaded Jessie to use it, is *very low* doses of HRT. Another alternative is raloxifen, an estrogen look-alike, which acts like estrogens in bone but does not stimulate the breasts or the uterus. These estrogen look-alikes are called SERMs (selective estrogen receptor modulators). Many of them are being developed and will be useful for older women who wish to avoid the side effects of estrogen. Chapter 17 is devoted to osteoporosis.

The message here is that older women need to be given hormones gradually and in lower doses so that the body gradually gets used to them. The good news is that even these lower doses can still have a worthwhile effect on bone density. In view of some reports suggesting that HRT should not be used for longer than five years, it may be that we should avoid for the present the long-term use of HRT. Some osteoporosis experts have suggested that HRT could be given to women in their sixties and seventies and continued long term to treat or prevent osteoporotic fractures in the hip and spine, but in my experience older women without any menopause symptoms are reluctant to take HRT because of potential side effects, such as bleeding and breast soreness, and risks such as potentiation of a breast cancer.

Two cases of the adverse side effects of HRT, especially the estrogen component, which throw the body out of physical balance have been presented above.

It should also be noted that in Australia it is the practice to give HRT continuously rather than cyclically (three weeks out of four). This is done to prevent cyclical bleeding, since most women do not want to go on having periods after menopause. It may be that continuous rather than cyclical estrogens, while keeping symptoms like hot flushes away, may leave no space for side effects to subside each month and thus increase the risk of some side effects such as bloating, breast soreness and mood swings. The answer to this is to keep doses low and for some women to use a cyclical pattern, if they will accept a monthly bleed for the sake of avoiding the estrogen build-up effect.

Recent concerns about the progestogen component of HRT perhaps increasing HRT risks such as breast cancer and clotting are not convincing, but have provoked fear among the women who have been on combination therapy to the point where many of these women have simply abandoned therapy and many of them have found no alternative that will give relief of symptoms such as hot flushes. Women on short-term therapy (less than five years) can be reassured that it is appropriate and safe.

We do not nowadays claim that HRT prevents or alleviates coronary artery disease or stroke. In the 1980s HRT *was* thought to be protective against heart attack and stroke. Many women were put on it for this reason alone, based on the observation that the incidence of heart attack in men is always greater than in women until women reach menopause. Then the rate of heart attack becomes similar in men and women. Since estrogen levels drop at menopause, lack of estrogen was thought to play a part in this increased risk. We now consider that lifestyle factors such as smoking, obesity, high cholesterol levels, high blood pressure and lack of exercise are the major risk factors for heart attack and stroke.

Giving HRT to a healthy, fit menopausal woman (called primary prevention) will not do anything positive for her heart, as her risk is already low. Giving HRT to unfit older women will not reduce cardiovascular risk either.

The HERS study (1998) showed an increased risk of cardiovascular disease (CVD) in women with heart disease given HRT for secondary prevention. These were older women who already had significant risk factors or had already had a heart attack or stroke.

The WHI study (2002), a chronic disease prevention trial supposedly of primary prevention of CVD, showed an increased risk.

Recent publications have emphasised that the timing of hormone therapy is very important as regards CVD outcomes, with perimenopausal and immediately postmenopausal women not being at increased risk, while those many years post-menopausal were more likely to have adverse events. This is crucial as HRT is used, conventionally, mainly for symptomatic women around the time of menopause.

Funding for a major study, the WISDOM study, which had enrolled many Australian women, has been withdrawn and the true answers to the absolute and long-term risks of HRT remain uncertain. The present advice is that HRT be prescribed for up to five years for menopause symptoms and not for protection from cardiovascular risk. For the long-term management of osteoporosis, medications other than HRT are now becoming available, as mentioned earlier, with the present cost of such drugs the only drawback to prescription.

The other aspect that needs to be considered is the emotional one. Too little estrogen makes moods sink. Too much produces irritability (as in the premenstrual syndrome). Therefore, in the woman who has had a hysterectomy (and therefore has no periods to mark the cycle), we must measure hormone levels to be sure whether the symptoms are due to menopause or not. There are so many other things happening around this time that we sometimes need to look to other causes for the emotional roller-coaster that some women find themselves riding. Medically, we need to get the hormone balance right. Emotionally, women also need to find a balance. This will be discussed in more detail in the final chapter.

Summary

- Loss of balance in a woman in midlife may be hormonal or emotional, or both.
- Balance is also required in prescribing medication – the needs of each woman have to be balanced against the possible side effects of the HRT.
- Long-term use of HRT is still being debated, but it appears that HRT can be safely given for periods up to five years.
- New forms of HRT helpful for symptoms in the post-menopausal woman and medications other than HRT for long-term management of osteoporosis are now available.
- Older women need to be given hormones gradually and in lower doses so that the body gradually gets used to them.

11

To bleed or not to bleed – that is the question

The desire of women to maintain the beneficial systemic effects of hormones on the quality and longevity of their lives has exposed them to the inevitable problems of endometrial bleeding.

SK Smith, *Progress in the Management of the Menopause*

The menopause is a point in time, the last menstrual period. It can only be truly diagnosed in retrospect when there has been no menstrual bleeding for twelve months. The ovaries have failed or are no longer responsive. Estrogen levels are falling and the lining of the uterus (the endometrium) is no longer stimulated, does not grow and therefore there is nothing to shed, so menstruation does not occur.

Some women think that this tissue, the endometrium, 'dies' after the menopause, but this is far from the truth. It is the amazing responsiveness of this tissue that leads to one of the most annoying side effects of using HRT – uterine bleeding. Feeding it with estrogens again, even after the lapse of many years, will make it grow and then it may have to bleed. This is why women in their sixties or seventies, who are sometimes given HRT even at this late age because of osteoporosis, may refuse to continue it. Not only do their breasts get sore, but also bleeding can occur after years of no bleeding. This is not welcome! Some women feel defined by their menstrual cycles and sincerely regret or even mourn their passing, but for most women the end of menstruation is a relief, especially if in the years preceding menopause – the premenopausal era – their periods have been heavy or painful or unpredictable. In pre-Pill days the end of menstruation was a relief because conception was no longer a problem.

The endometrium is one of the most remarkable tissues in the body. Each month it has to build up under the influence of estrogen, and then become secretory (i.e. nourishing) under the influence of progesterone, so that it is ready to receive an embryo, and it must shed down to the most basal layer if pregnancy does not occur. One of my poetic teachers of long ago described menstruation as 'the tears of the disappointed uterus', weeping because it had no baby to nourish. Menstruation represents the failure of reproduction, but the success of contraception.

> One of my poetic teachers … described menstruation as 'the tears of the disappointed uterus', weeping because it had no baby to nourish.

Estrogen makes the endometrial cells grow and divide (the estrogens used in HRT also produce growth of the endometrial cells). Progesterone changes the cells into less active, secretory, or nourishing, cells and this stops the rapid growth induced by the estrogens. As women approach menopause progesterone secretion is often diminished or absent, so periods become heavier because of the unopposed estrogen effect. This is called menorrhagia or *dysfunctional bleeding*.

Menstruation is not what nature really intended for the female body. Nature would have women pregnant or lactating (breastfeeding) for most of their reproductive lives and thus menstruating only sporadically.

When HRT was first introduced, in the mid-sixties in the USA, estrogen only (Premarin) was given. Women did not mind bleeding again, but when abnormal bleeding occurred and curettage was performed it was found that this estrogen-only stimulation over time increased the incidence of endometrial cancer sevenfold (the usual incidence is one in a thousand, so seven cases per thousand was not a large *overall* number, but it certainly was noticeable and initially frightening). Adding a progestogen to the estrogen stopped uterine cancer happening, so these days, if a woman still has her uterus, HRT will consist of an estrogen plus a progestogen. Cyclic therapy with estrogen for four weeks and progestogen for only two weeks will reproduce cyclical bleeding. The latter is the way that HRT is often given in the USA. Most women prefer to have no bleeding at all, so in Australia it is common to give continuous combined HRT, i.e. a fixed dose of estrogen and progestogen without a break.

However, the endometrium, being the sensitive tissue that it is, often has other ideas, so that in the first six to twelve months of the continuous type of HRT 'nuisance' bleeding is not rare. By 'nuisance' we mean that there is no pathology present and therefore the bleeding is not dangerous, but it is an annoyance, especially as it is so variable and unpredictable. Because of this, many women will give up therapy (which is otherwise helping them) because such bleeding is unacceptable. The other 'nuisance' bleeding is flooding, which can occur before menopause due to lack of progesterone. I am continually amazed by some women's forbearance with this flooding. In some women it leads to hysterectomy, but many others grimly put up with it even though they run short of iron and are anaemic and tired and often housebound by it.

Marlena is aged 49. For the last two years her periods have been increasingly heavy, so that for at least the first three days of each period she is afraid to leave the house. She passes huge clots, which make her feel faint and are often accompanied by pains that remind her of labour pains. She has a husband and two children and she also works full-time as a teacher.

When I first saw her she was extremely pale, her blood count was very low (i.e. she was anaemic) and her blood iron level was extremely low. Her own doctor had started her on a course of iron injections, as she had been unable to take iron tablets by mouth because of the resultant constipation.

An ultrasound showed that she had large fibroids with one of these impinging on the cavity of the uterus. Most fibroids are *within* the wall of the uterus. They do not actually *cause* the bleeding but are a sign that estrogen levels are high because estrogens can make fibroids grow. The bleeding is caused by the excessive build-up of the endometrium under strong estrogen stimulation but without enough progesterone being available to prevent this. We call these cycles 'anovulatory', meaning there is no ovulation; therefore no progesterone is produced in the ovary. This hormonal imbalance we call 'dysfunctional' and the bleeding that results is also called 'dysfunctional'. Cancer of the endometrium is not common at this time but is always investigated by dilatation and curettage (D&C) if there is any suspicion of this. When a fibroid impinges on the cavity of the uterus, though, it may cause extra bleeding from its surface. I usually recommend hysterectomy for this situation.

Marlena was unwilling to have a hysterectomy despite the fact that her bleeding was potentially life threatening. She was afraid of the operative risks, particularly the anaesthetic, and she also felt that to lose her uterus was to lose what defined her as a woman. These were difficult objections to overcome!

I suggested that she take the oral contraceptive pill to control her cycle. She objected to this because of possible side effects. My argument that the side effects of the pill were probably minor compared with the risks of the flooding did not convince her. So I gave her some progestogen tablets, in a fairly high dose, to be taken from the 12th day of the cycle to the 25th day (the first day of bleeding is day one of a cycle). She had some relief from this in the next two cycles, and then the bleeding again turned into a flood. I then gave her a medication called Danazol, which we often use in women who have endometriosis. It works by switching off the menstrual cycle. This worked well but because of the cost she could only use it for six months. She kept hoping that menopause would rescue her, but I had to point out that she had probably another three or four years of menstrual cycles to endure.

Finally, after coming off the Danazol and again having huge flooding, she agreed to a hysterectomy. This was done via the laparoscope so that there was no abdominal wound to cause pain. She was surprised that she was able to go home on the fourth day after the operation. She has recovered so quickly and feels so well now that her blood count has improved that she has finally admitted that it was the right treatment and that she should have had it sooner. Her ovaries were left in so that she is not truly menopausal. Her periods have ceased but the ovaries are still producing hormones.

Lara, aged 48, has 3 sons – the youngest is 11.This young lad has been most concerned about his mother who is having flooding. At one stage when she was marooned in the bathroom, unable to come out, he knocked at the door and offered her a Band-Aid and a blanket! She feels that the girl that he marries will be looked after and lucky. Lara took an oral contraceptive pill which controlled the flooding by switching off her own cycle. She will probably not need a hysterectomy as menopause is likely within the next three years and she does not have any pathology such as fibroids. Her bleeding is dysfunctional.

Hysterectomy has been called 'the unkindest cut of all', with apologies to Shakespeare. It is not an acceptable option for many women because the negative aspects have been widely reported and the positive aspects dismissed. One of my patients told me that her husband, after she had had a hysterectomy, made her feel that she had a 'use-by date printed on her forehead'!

In the past, hysterectomy was thought to lead to sexual dysfunction because of removal of the cervix (the neck of the womb), but few people believe this now. It was also thought to cause psychological problems because some women felt that the presence of the uterus defined them as women and that its removal led to a loss and grief reaction.

The good news is that there are other ways to control heavy bleeding, for example, ablation of the endometrium (burning off the lining with microwaves) or embolisation of the arteries feeding the fibroid, causing the arteries to close with clot and thus starving the fibroid so that it shrinks. One of my patients asked me 'Do I really need my uterus? It is rather like carrying around an empty handbag!' She gratefully exchanged her heavy, painful bleeding for a hysterectomy.

It is necessary to say that menstrual disorders and dysfunctions are the inevitable result of modern woman's attempts to deny her reproductive potential.

Bleeding that occurs after periods have ceased altogether is called postmenopausal bleeding and is one of the main reasons why women will not take, or have to give up taking, HRT. However, if the two hormones, estrogen and progestogen, are taken on a continuous basis, we can give reassurance that this combination of hormones will produce little, if any, endometrial stimulation and therefore no bleeding. There is also no cancer risk.

Because the endometrium is so exquisitely responsive to hormones, in practice it is not easy to achieve a state of no bleeding, especially within the first twelve months of menopause. But as long as women are warned of this, most are prepared to put up with it. New combination patches and tablets are claimed to be the ideal combinations, but in practice the likelihood of breakthrough bleeding remains high. It is usually nuisance bleeding, as explained previously, although an ultrasound to check on the thickness of the lining is usually needed and sometimes dilatation and curettage of the uterus has to be done. All this makes it costly and time consuming to make a diagnosis so as to exclude cancer or other pathology. The Mirena IUD is now proving useful to control unwanted bleeding. It contains a progestogen which counteracts the effect of estrogen on the endometrium.

Fortunately we now have an alternative to conventional HRT in the form of tibolone (see also Chapters 4 and 10), which is what I call 'Clayton's HRT'. It has the advantages of hormones without breast or endometrial stimulation. Thus it does not usually cause bleeding nor does it cause breast activity. Why is this not used more often instead of HRT if it appears so effective? Some women say they have found it less effective for hot flushes and other menopausal symptoms. It is also more expensive than HRT.

So, to answer this chapter's question, 'To bleed or not to bleed?', not to bleed is definitely preferable and can usually be attained. And, of course, the cause of abnormal bleeding in a woman on HRT is usually an imbalance of hormones. The answer to our recurrent question, 'Is it me or my hormones?' is a definite 'It's your hormones'.

Summary

- When a woman is given estrogen, she may experience the side effect of uterine bleeding.
- Estrogen makes the endometrial cells grow and divide; progesterone stops the rapid growth.
- As women approach menopause and their progesterone diminishes their periods may become heavier. This is known as dysfunctional bleeding.
- As most women prefer not to bleed, a fixed dose of estrogen and progestogen taken continuously is recommended, although this can still lead to nuisance bleeding or flooding.
- For health and psychological reasons, it is sometimes necessary for women to have a hysterectomy to put an end to flooding, although there are two other possible effective treatments.
- Today, an effective alternative to conventional HRT is available called tibolone, which does not cause bleeding or breast activity.

12

I'm running out of restaurants –
the hot flush

Bello e il rossore, ma e incommodo qualche volta.
(The blush is beautiful, but is sometimes inconvenient.)

Carlo Goldoni (1707–1793)

When Theresa made the statement, as we started our interview, that she was 'running out of restaurants', I thought she was going to tell me a *When Harry met Sally* type of story – that there were some restaurants she and her partner could not go back to because of their sexual exploits (or perhaps her violent mood swings causing a fair amount of broken crockery!) No, my imagination had it wrong. She was literally running out the doors of restaurants because she was overwhelmed by hot flushes and had become intensely claustrophobic.

Women who have never experienced hot flushes need to be very careful about judging those who have severe, frequent flushes (or 'flashes' as they say in the USA). These can be extremely debilitating. I have known women whose social life has been destroyed by them, especially if the flushes are followed by drenching sweating of the head and neck. We still do not know exactly why flushes occur. They are clearly related to estrogen deficiency and also to release of the ovary-stimulating hormones from the pituitary gland, especially the luteinising hormone (LH), which normally triggers ovulation. They are worse in fair or red-skinned women and in hot climates. They will usually subside within two to five years but some women will still have flushes in their sixties.

At the International Congress on Menopause in Stockholm in 1993, Drs Ginsberg and Hardiman presented a fascinating paper – 'The menopausal hot flush: facts and fancies' – from which I have derived some of the following information.

Flushes were first described and named in the eighteenth century. A French physician called them 'bouffes de chaleur' (puffs of heat), and by the nineteenth century, women suffering these puffs of heat were warned to avoid large gatherings and heated rooms.

An English physician named Tilt noted in 1858 that nearly 50 percent of the 500 women in his study of menopausal women had significant hot flushes. This is the same figure noted in all the recent large studies of menopause. He noted that menopausal women in general seemed to 'generate more heat, and tended to leave windows and doors open and that they were specific complications of the menopause'.

Modern studies measuring skin temperature and peripheral blood flow, particularly to the head and arms, have shown that *flushes are not the same as blushes*. Certain women may be more susceptible to both and stress is a precipitating factor for both. Germaine Greer, in her book, *The Change*, says: 'the process that causes the blood vessels in the surface of the skin to dilate is similar to the mechanism that makes some of us go hot with embarrassment and go red'. She has no more sympathy for the woman tormented by hot flushes than the Victorian doctors who recommended cold baths and avoidance of hot places. There are still many unbelievers. It is hard for those women suffering distress and needing to run out of restaurants to be so put down.

In the middle of the last century barbiturates were prescribed to keep women calm and hopefully switch off the flushes. These were singularly unsuccessful in that they switched off the woman but not the flushes.

Men may also have hot flushes if they have both testicles removed, e.g. for prostatic cancer. So the *mechanism of flushes is not simply estrogen deficiency* but a complex cascade of events involving the pituitary and the hypothalamus (the area above the pituitary which acts as a neural network centre). However, *estrogen therapy is far and away the most effective therapy that we have at present to control hot flushes.* Many other things have been tried, e.g. small doses of antihypertensive agents such as clonidine. Natural therapies are not very effective for severe flushing, though plant 'estrogens' may help with mild flushes. Incidentally, plants do not have estrogens as women do. The substances we call estrogens in plants are really to ward off invaders, not to provide for reproduction. Recently, certain types of antidepressant medications in small doses have been shown to effectively relieve hot flushes for some women. This may be related to the effects of such drugs to improve mood and sleeping patterns (they act on the neural centre as described above).

Recently, certain types of antidepressant medications in small doses have been shown to effectively relieve hot flushes for some women.

You may wonder why we are spending a whole chapter on this one symptom. Hot flushes are far and away the most common symptom of menopause and can be extremely debilitating and distressing. They are often dismissed by those who haven't experienced them as being inconsequential. They are treated with derision and are a subject of sly laughter. I had personal experience of this. A surgical menopause, removal of uterus and both ovaries, at age 43, precipitated menopause for me and the hot flushes were overwhelming. And it is not just the flush itself that is disturbing but also the feeling of coldness and shivering that follows. There is also a feeling of confusion. I was a university clinical lecturer at this time, teaching fifth-year medical students, and I often lost the thread of my lecture and found it hard to recover my composure. I had a fund of jokes which I could usually rely on to bring the students back when their attention was faltering, but I could not even tell these without losing the punch line. It was a time of great embarrassment for me so that blushing often followed the flushing. Again I stress the point that flushing and blushing are separate entities and disagree with Germaine Greer who says that the mechanisms are similar.

Drs Ginsberg and Hardiman noted that 'Women who flush tend to be more heat intolerant than others. Heat intolerance is present even when they are not actually flushing. They are hot when they are doing their housework, they are hot at night and they may even sleep on top of the bedcovers. It has been claimed that women who flush frequently have higher blood pressures than those who do not.'

These doctors studied a group of women and showed that there were changes in other aspects of cardiovascular function in the 'flushers'. Therefore the flush may be only one manifestation of a more widespread disturbance in cardiovascular function after the menopause. However, it was disappointing to find that medications such as clonidine (which normally control blood pressure by stopping the constriction of blood vessels) did not relieve flushes as expected. There are no suitable animal models. Rats do not flush or blush, though the skin temperature of their tails changes with varying levels of hormones at oestrus and this seems to be more pronounced as they age. As far as I know, no-one has ever reported on rats running out of restaurants because their tails are on fire!

'My thermostat is broken', one of my patients reported to me, and I think that she is near to the mark. The thermoregulatory centre in the hypothalamus is responding to confusing messages and making inappropriate responses. The typical area of flushing is the head and the neck. Many women become bright red in these areas but others have the feeling without anything to show for it; in other words, it is invisible to others.

Jane came to me because she was acutely embarrassed by her facial and neck redness. She had been having episodic flushes. These had quietened down with estrogen therapy but the redness remained. Her blood pressure was normal. She has a fair complexion, typical of someone born in the north of England. Her mother always had a very high colour, which was also worse after menopause. I sent her for a battery of other hormone tests, since hormones inducing redness and flushing may be produced in the gut or other areas of the body. All the tests were negative. She has now been referred to a skin specialist who will consider laser therapy to the affected superficial blood vessels.

Elizabeth is now 63. She went through menopause, without many problems, at the age of 54. She had moderately severe hot flushes, which were well controlled by HRT. She ceased this three years ago. She is now troubled by sweating of the face and neck. It is so severe that she is embarrassed to go out. Her hair is always dripping wet. She went back on HRT but the problem remains, despite increasing doses of HRT to the point of producing breast soreness. She had heard of a hypnotist who claimed success in treating excess sweating. His treatment worked initially but then the problem returned. She has a condition called hyperhidrosis, which simply means excessive sweating. I referred her to a vascular surgeon who has performed a laparoscopic sympathectomy, a procedure to sever the autonomic or sympathetic nerves in the axilla (armpits). This has been entirely successful, though there has been an increase in sweating in the lower half of her body, as expected. This she can cope with, unlike the head sweating, which was so socially embarrassing.

Many people would agree with the psychosocial researchers who suggest that 'the assumption that menopause is a universal experience at any level, biological, physiological or social, should be subjected to serious questioning'. Germaine Greer certainly seems to hold this view, though in a recent interview she confessed to using hormones herself, including, briefly, testosterone. Some psychosocial researchers suggest that many of the symptoms which women expect to have and which have been attributed to menopause in the medical literature are *components in a stereotype of menopausal women rather then the actual experience in the majority of women*.

It is true that reported symptoms vary. For example, those of Japanese women differ markedly from those reported by North American women. It is also true that HRT has not been generally available to women in Japan whereas it has been to North American women, so that in ordinary medical practice in Japan no relevant questions are asked. I don't want to talk Japanese women into having hot flushes but I would like to think that there is some help available for those who do have them. Madame Albery, a Japanese woman, spoke on this subject at the 1996 International Menopause Congress in Sydney. She claimed that many women in modern Japan have suffered silently, and she has founded the Amarant Society, which has the motto, 'My body, my life, my choice'.

I am not really concerned, as a practising gynaecologist, to determine the exact incidence of symptoms among the total of women I see in my practice. What I want to do is to hear their individual stories and to relieve symptoms if they are troublesome. Hot flushes can be devastating for some women, making social life impossible. To me, to paraphrase the wise eccentric poet Gertrude Stein, 'a hot flush is a hot flush is a hot flush'. Let's not try to explain flushes away, or say they don't happen, and then, perhaps, we will have fewer women running out of restaurants!

This chapter, more than any other, illustrates how potent hormones are and how a lack of them can produce real deficiency symptoms, hot flushes being the most obvious of these. Hot flushes are not particularly related to a woman's emotional make-up. Fair-skinned women may have more noticeable flushing (and blushing) than those with olive complexions, as we have mentioned, but the latter may have worse sweats. Hot flushes are truly hormonal and, despite all attempts to find some other remedy, estrogen therapy is the only known inhibitor of them. For menopausal women, hot flushes *are* due to 'hormones' (actually the *lack* of hormones) rather than the personality or 'me'.

Summary

- Hot flushes are by far the most common symptom of menopause and can cause great distress to women.
- Hot flushes are related to estrogen deficiency and to the release of ovary-stimulating hormones.
- Blushes and flushes are different.
- Flushes may be followed by coldness and shivering and may be accompanied by confusion.
- Estrogen therapy is the most effective remedy to date for controlling hot flushes.

13

I really miss my mind –
the hereafter syndrome

O the mind, mind has mountains; cliffs of fall
Frightful, sheer, no-man-fathomed. Hold them cheap
May who ne'er hung there.

Gerard Manley Hopkins (1844–1889)

The classic joke about a menopausal woman is that she walks among the shelves in a supermarket, stands there somewhat dazed and wonders 'What am I here after?' Hence this midlife memory loss has been dubbed 'the hereafter syndrome'.

Here are some verses given to me by one of my patients. She said she could have written this herself:

Just a line to say I'm living,
That I'm not amongst the dead,
Though I'm getting more forgetful
And mixed up in the head.

I've got used to my arthritis,
To my dentures I'm resigned,

I can cope with my bifocals,
But — ye gods — I miss my mind!

Sometimes I can't remember
When I'm standing by the stair,
If I should go up for something,
Or I've just come down from there?

And before the fridge so often
My mind is full of doubt,
Now did I put some food away,
Or come to take some out?

If it's not my turn to write dear
I hope you won't get sore,
I think I may have written
And don't want to be a bore.

So remember I do love you,
And wish that you lived near,
And now it's time to mail this
And to say goodbye, my dear.

At last I stand before the mailbox
And my face — it sure is red.
Instead of posting this to you
I've opened it instead!

Many women ask, 'Am I going crazy?' and 'Is it me or is it my hormones?' The question that carries the most dread of all is, 'Do I have Alzheimer's?'

Vanessa, a delightful woman with an engaging smile and a wicked sense of humour, told me, 'My Mum says that I was born with Alzheimer's.' She said it had always been such a standard family joke that to become more forgetful at this time of life was no big deal for her. Her outlook was positive and refreshing, rather like the famous Colette who said, 'You will do foolish things, but do them with enthusiasm.'

Most women can be reassured that they do not have incipient or actual Alzheimer's. In fact, if someone asks the question, the answer is usually no, because someone with Alzheimer's does not usually ask. Other people ask it for them. The true sadness of this disease is the suffering of the loved ones who see the ravages being wrought. After the initial stage of awareness the patient is no longer aware of the changes happening. The description of the gradual dismantling of an intelligent mind, and the pain endured by her husband, is told vividly in the story of the brilliant English writer, Iris Murdoch, who died in 2002.

The forgetfulness that happens in midlife is only partly related to hormone deficiency and affects mainly the short-term memory.

One of her early novels had the strangely appropriate and prescient title, *A Severed Head*. There is no evidence that Alzheimer's is directly linked to hormones, but HRT may delay the onset of some symptoms.

The forgetfulness that happens in midlife is only partly related to hormone deficiency and affects mainly the short-term memory. It is related to mental and physical tiredness and leads to loss of self-confidence, which feeds back to become confusion and embarrassment. So there is a whole cascade of events which further sap self-confidence. Reassurance usually restores equilibrium. HRT is most helpful when hot flushes are a problem and sleep is disturbed. There is some evidence that estrogens may improve short-term memory.

In fact, many of the symptoms at midlife are psychosocial rather than hormonal. As will be discussed in Chapter 16 on depression, no increase in the incidence of major depression or mental functioning associated with natural menopause has been demonstrated. Women who are depressed before menopause may find, though, that it gets worse at this time.

My great friend of 50 years, Liz, always delightfully vague (she went through menopause, as through every other passage in her life without particularly noting what was happening), passes off these momentary glitches in memory as 'senior moments'. I do remember that many years ago she took her children to the beach and then wandered off home leaving them there. Fortunately, they were old enough to find their way home without her and so used to her absentmindedness that they were not too fazed when she asked them where they had been! It would be no good giving Liz hormones. She would never remember to take them.

Hormone deficiency, particularly estrogen deficiency, has been shown to result in some changes in mood and learning ability, as well as in memory. Many studies done in the USA show that women who are on HRT are less likely to develop dementing illness and that estrogens may have beneficial effects on verbal memory; however, scientists are saying that a long-term prospective trial is needed before doctors should put women on long-term therapy for the *sole* purpose of improving brain function. Previous studies may have been skewed because present estrogen users, especially in the USA, tend to be of a different social class and higher education than non-users.

Sally came to see me accompanied by her husband, Tom. He shepherded her in and started to take over the interview. She is 56. Menopause was gradual, starting at 53. She had sleep disturbance and many hot flushes, but because her mother had breast cancer she was loathe to take HRT. She had been working as a florist but now found it difficult to cope with some aspects of her work, particularly adding up money. Colleagues were irritated by her slowness. She therefore, regretfully, left her job. At home she annoyed her husband and daughter by losing things. She had no confidence on the phone. She was inclined to panic and hang up if it was business or the bank manager. Her husband kept telling her not to be so stupid and, as he was telling me this story, he was glancing at her angrily. She ducked her head as if to duck the question also. I tried to talk to her directly but she deferred to Tom and smiled faintly even though her demeanour otherwise was withdrawn. She was not clinically depressed.

Clinically, Sally has early Alzheimer's Disease. I started her on HRT mainly for her hot flushes, and she had a full assessment for her mild dementia, which confirmed the diagnosis of early Alzheimer's. Her husband and her daughter did not want to accept the diagnosis. I tried to talk to Tom after I had sent Sally back to the waiting room, where she sat with a vacant look on her face and did not attempt to read any of the magazines. Tom was angry – with me, and with Sally, and with the world in general. 'I've got a busy life. I can't look after a wife who is behaving stupidly. She will just have to pull herself together and learn to cope better.' I just listened to him. What was there to say or do?

Three months later, Sally came back to see me. This time she came into my office alone. Her daughter had driven her to my rooms, but she wanted to come in to see me by herself. She was still rather vague, but her affect was different. She seemed happier and much more in touch with her surroundings. Her daughter confirmed this. Tom had settled down too, but he still thinks that the diagnosis is wrong and that all Sally needs is a good pep talk and some HRT.

Sally's dementia will continue but it is possible that the HRT will slow the process.

Many other women present with mild memory loss, fuzziness in the head and an inability to think clearly. 'Will hormones help?' is the common question they ask.

It is important to get a clear picture of what else is happening in their life at this time. There are often enormous emotional, if not physical, demands being made. Hot flushes may be disturbing sleep and it is well known that the lack of sleep results in muddled thinking and mental fuzziness. A trial of HRT is well worthwhile, as was demonstrated in Sally's case. There is no doubt that a woman's self-esteem is of immense importance to her wellbeing. If this is battered she may be unable to function mentally or sexually. However, on the whole, HRT cannot restore the slowing down of some of our mental processes, which happens with age.

There is growing evidence that testosterone, the main male hormone, has protective effects on some brain functions, mainly concentration and mood. It can be worthwhile measuring testosterone if symptoms such as lowered mood, lack of concentration and lack of libido are prominent. The use of testosterone replacement in women will be discussed in more detail in Chapter 21.

Summary

- Many women fear the onset of Alzheimer's Disease when they experience the forgetfulness and fuzziness that can occur during midlife. However, if you are able to ask, 'Do I have Alzheimer's?', the answer is generally no.
- Forgetfulness is partly related to hormone deficiency and partly to mental and physical tiredness. HRT can help if hot flushes and sleep disturbance are present.
- Again, it is important to assess a woman's total history as emotional factors may also be a cause of memory loss and mental fuzziness.
- There is some evidence that the male hormone, testosterone, may have some effect on concentration and mood.

14

I'm sick and tired of being sick and tired!

Life is one long process of getting tired.

Samuel Butler (1835–1902)

My mother wrote this little set of verses down for me when she was going through her own menopause and I was a young doctor who had not been taught anything about menopause. 'The end of periods' was the definition we were given, implying that no treatment was needed. Hormone replacement was not considered since it was not available.

Here lies a poor woman, who always was tired,
She lived in a house where help wasn't hired.
The last words she said were: 'Dear friends, I am going
Where washing ain't wanted, nor sweeping nor sewing;
And everything there is exact to my wishes,
For when folk don't eat, there's no washing of dishes.

'In heaven loud anthems forever are ringing,
But having no voice, I'll keep clear of the singing.

Don't mourn for me now; don't mourn for me never,
I'm going to do nothing for ever and ever.'

My mother was very tired at this time. She was not sleeping well and she was irritable.

Tiredness and sickness are usually physical, but we need to look at the emotional aspects also. And we need to ask more questions. What, or perhaps who, is making you tired?

'A woman's work is never done', lamented our mothers and grandmothers. It is still true today despite labour-saving devices. Housework has not yet been abolished. It has changed its nature, but it is still housework, or more correctly family work, which is largely unpaid and seldom applauded. **A man does not often do a woman's work, even though increasingly women are performing men's work.**

My friend, Susan Maushart, writes tellingly about this in her book, *Wifework*:

> Eva, a friend of mine living in an all-male household, is sick and tired that so much is expected of her and so little help is given. The Christmas and New Year period always stretches her to the limit because of the cleaning up afterwards. Her tiredness is largely related to the resentment she feels. She is at menopause but has plenty of energy for the things she wants to do, but being the family drudge tries her patience and her stamina. Her relationship is threatened by her resentment and her husband continues to be demanding and cannot understand her reactions.

A man does not often do a woman's work, even though increasingly women are performing men's work. Some who choose to do this find that they are expected to be the chief family houseworker and caregiver as well.

Germaine Greer in *The Whole Woman* has much to say on this subject that confirms the dissatisfaction that so many of my patients express with their role as it is at midlife:

> Women are the labouring sex. All over the world women do the heavy, mindless repetitive labour. Comparison of a woman's workload with a man's is difficult because a good deal of women's effort is not even recognised as work. Only a fraction of the work that women do produces an income. The rest is done because somebody has to do it, if life is to be livable.
>
> Male animals are conspicuously less busy than females, yet somehow the human male has convinced the human female that he, not she, is the worker. Leisure is a masculine privilege.

As Greer says, in other species it is also the females who are naturally busy (worker bees) and the males who do little (drones). During my seven years as an obstetrician–gynaecologist in the highlands of New Guinea in the 1960s, before the country was independent, I saw women become prematurely old (if they survived childbirth) because of the rigours of their work. Men sat around telling stories or perhaps preparing to fight with a neighbouring tribe, but certainly were not involved in food growing, gathering or cooking. They also took little part in childcare. When the country became independent in 1973 many men found it hard to make the transition from drones to workers.

One of the most delightful, if eccentric, women I have ever read about was reported in our national newspaper, *The Australian*, in a story headed, 'Woman's work is always done in a self-clean house'. Driven by her hatred of housework, this 81-year-old American woman had developed a self-cleaning house. Since she completed the house in 1990, she has been trying to market her inventions with little success. Maybe not many people feel so strongly about housework. I like her story, but perhaps there is a middle road, and there may be other causes for tiredness attributed to too much housework, as we shall see below.

Wendy's first words to me when I asked her to tell her story were, 'Every night I feel that I just fall over the line'. Wendy is 52. Her periods 'went out with a bang' six months ago. She had flooding and was given an oral contraceptive pill to control this. The bleeding settled but her tiredness remained. She is having flushes, is sleeping poorly, and has little sex drive, but her major problem is the extreme tiredness. She has three children in their twenties. They are all male. Two are working, but the youngest is on the dole and has decided that he is not interested in getting a job. He has kicked a drug habit but she still feels concerned that he may go back to it. They all still live at home. Her husband has a poorly paid job so Wendy has also worked outside the home for most of her married life. She is on her feet all day. She has no time for formal exercise and she has no leisure time.

There were several physical causes for the fatigue. Blood tests showed a low iron count, low estrogens and borderline thyroid levels. All these were treated. Three months later, Wendy was less tired physically, but was still 'just falling over the line' and her sex drive was still very low. She was not clinically depressed, but her mood was one of resignation. There was little joy in her life. She could not imagine any change in her circumstances being possible. She *is* mildly depressed but I don't think antidepressants will help much. She is trapped by circumstances, which seem to be beyond her control.

Wendy exemplifies the lot of many women who feel trapped, helpless, sad, unheard and unvalidated. A woman's need for self-esteem and validation is emerging as a common theme for emotional health at midlife. HRT cannot fix emotional tiredness and the circumstances that cause this.

I saw Wendy again a bit later. After an episode of chest pain she had been found to have a heart problem, which none of us had suspected or detected! So she was unvalidated medically as well as emotionally. As a gynaecologist I am not expert in cardiology, but even a general physician had overlooked her heart problem because it had not presented in a classical way. Wendy has had much of her lost vigour restored by appropriate treatment and regaining physical strength has lifted her mood.

There is a major lesson here again – consider the *whole* woman, not just her circumstances, the amount of housework she has to do, and her possible hormone deficiencies.

Summary

- At midlife many women get tired. While this may be related to menopause, it can also have an emotional or physical cause.
- Women do work hard, sometimes these days doing both housework and work outside the home.
- Women's need for self-esteem and validation are important for emotional health in midlife.

15

The way we were –
a weighty problem

I'm not overweight, just nine inches too short.

Shelley Winters

'A man is as old as he feels and a woman as old as she looks' proclaims a nineteenth-century proverb. This is true for many people and can provoke marital disaster as the male partner maintains good skin texture and general fitness, while his wife starts to sag in all the wrong places, gains weight, and may also have menopause symptoms such as flushes, sleeplessness and a decline in sexual feelings. Sophia Loren, who appears ageless, has maintained fitness without fatness so there must be some hope for others. She claims: 'All you see I owe to spaghetti'; however, I don't think that living on a high carbohydrate diet will keep the rest of us slim.

A recent circular letter on the Internet tells us about 'The Ages of Women':

Age 8: Looks at herself and sees Cinderella, Sleeping Beauty, etc.
Age 15: Looks at herself and sees Cinderella/Sleeping Beauty/class

leader; or if she is PMS-ing sees fat/pimples/ugly and says 'Mum, I can't go to school looking like this.'

Age 20: Looks at herself and sees too fat/too thin/too short/too tall/too straight/too curly, but decides she can go anyway.

Age 30: Looks at herself and sees too fat/too thin/too short/too tall/too straight/too curly, but decides she doesn't have time to fix it and goes anyway.

Age 40: Looks at herself and sees too fat/too thin/too tall/too short/too tall/too straight/too curly, but says, 'At least I'm clean' and she goes anyway.

Age 50: Looks at herself and says, 'I am', and goes wherever she wants to go.

Age 60: Looks at herself and reminds herself of all the people in the world who can't even see themselves in a mirror any more. Goes out and conquers the world.

Age 70: Looks at herself and sees wisdom, laughter and ability. Goes out and enjoys life.

Age 80: Doesn't bother to look. Just puts on a red hat and goes out to participate in the world.

Age 90: Can't see but doesn't worry about it!

I'm not so sure that women are as accepting of physical change as this suggests. Of course, it is not possible to preserve our youthful physical characteristics into old age. Even Gypsy Rose Lee acknowledged that we droop with age. She said 'I have everything now that I had twenty years ago – except now it's all lower.' Most of us regret these changes even as we laugh ruefully about them! So many women I see feel that they are no longer attractive to others. They hate to see themselves in the mirror. They no longer feel sexy. One said to me that she no longer puts her glasses on when getting dressed as she can't bear how she looks.

It would be nice to think that, as we aged, we would care less about how we look and what others think, but we do care. Even my great friend,

Liz, admits that it is hard for her, at 71, to see a gorgeous hunk of man who does not even give her a second glance. Looking back wistfully she remembers when she usually got that second glance. The wonderful actress, Katharine Hepburn, claimed not to care about appearance and ageing. She said, 'I have no romantic feelings about age. Either you are interesting at any age or you are not. There is nothing particularly interesting about being old, or being young, for that matter.'

Some women spend large amounts of money on cosmetics, cosmetic surgery, shaping-up courses, diets, vitamins and

> Gypsy Rose Lee ... said 'I have everything now that I had twenty years ago – except now it's all lower.'

herbals. Physical fitness is desirable, of course, and it can help to prevent osteoporosis, but concentration on repair of the physical body is sometimes undertaken without due thought for mental and spiritual growth. 'Old age is not an illness', says American writer May Sarton, 'it is a timeless ascent. As power diminishes we grow toward the light.'

We all want to look good on the outside as well as feeling good on the inside. A major stress is the change in shape. Our breasts sag and get fatter. We bulge in all the wrong places. We lose our waists. We gain weight, or we remain the same weight and change shape! Is weight gain inevitable? We have all known, forever it seems, that there is something laughingly called 'the middle age spread'. It turns out to be true. It happens with age and it happens in the middle. One of the reasons that some women try to avoid HRT is that they have been told that HRT may cause weight gain. There is no scientific proof that the metabolic rate decreases after menopause unless there is some other factor present such as low thyroid hormone levels. Most doctors do check thyroid function in their menopausal patients. The bottom line is: women are not eating more but the weight does go on in middle age. So what is the cause?

Frances is now 53. A year ago her periods dwindled away and now she is having hot flushes and is sleeping poorly. She has gained 5 kilograms in weight, mostly around the middle. She was given combination HRT but ceased it after 3 months. It certainly helped the flushes but made her breasts increase in size, and she blames the HRT for the weight gain. She used to play tennis, but this at present increases her hot flushes. Because she is tired in the mornings after a restless night, she has not been walking three or four mornings a week as she used to do. Her sex drive is disappearing as well. She is an attractive woman, but does not feel good about herself any more. She agreed to try HRT again but this time in a lower dose, using a low dose patch as her estrogen and a small dose of a progestogen. This was enough to settle the flushes and increase her energy. She started playing tennis again, reduced fat and carbohydrate in her diet and lost the extra weight, as well as changing shape. When she started to feel better about herself her sex drive improved also.

Scientific studies of the effect of HRT on weight deny that HRT causes weight gain.

The PEPI (Postmenopausal Estrogen/Progestin Interval) trial reported in the *Journal of the American Medical Association* in 1996 was designed to find out if HRT offered some protection against the occurrence of heart attack and stroke. Incidentally, it showed that the women who gained most weight during this three-year study were those *not* on HRT! Yet many women know that when they went on the pill in the past, and if they use HRT now, they do feel bloated, their breasts may get heavier, and they thicken up around the middle. Reducing the dose of hormones *can* be helpful. Estrogens can also cause a problem with fluid retention. Taking hormones cyclically, rather than continuously, may be better as this may allow the weight to decrease at the end of the cycle – just as it does in the menstrual cycle. Unfortunately, cyclic HRT will produce bleeding again, and in the week off hormones the hot flushes may recur.

The better way to manage the weight problem is to change your diet. As well as decreasing fat intake, it is necessary to cut down on carbohydrates. There has been a big swing away from the high fat diets that my generation lived on, but often there has been a compensatory rise in carbohydrates. To eliminate carbohydrates altogether is not possible and is not healthy. Balance is needed and a good dietitian can help you.

Exercise is the other key. We have all become too used to wheels rather than walking. Remembering that exercise is also good for our bones and our arteries should spur us on.

Joy is now well named, but she was anything but joyful when I first met her. She was sent to me because she was depressed and overweight and she felt that HRT had made her worse. She had reasons to be less than joyful. Her husband was having an affair with a young woman in his office, and when Joy found out he had mocked her and told her he was leaving.

He told her that she was fat and ugly and no good in bed. Joy had given up her own career to have her children and support her husband. The children were successful and really did not need her any longer. There came a day when she caught sight of herself in the mirror and wondered who it was. Sagging skin, shapeless figure, dry hair, and lifeless sad eyes: she suddenly saw how she had let herself go. Her mother was mildly demented and had Joy running around after her, so Joy had less and less social life and no life of her own. She was shocked when she realised all this.

I sent Joy to a therapist who could help her look for the one she had lost. She enrolled at a gym and went to see a dietitian. Six months later, Joy came back to see me. She was smartly dressed and slimmer, but the most notable thing was the light in her eyes. Her self-esteem had risen.

Actor Jacqueline Bisset says: 'Character contributes to beauty. It fortifies a woman as her youth fades. A mode of conduct, a standard of courage, discipline, fortitude and integrity, can do a great deal to make a woman beautiful.'

Change of shape, increase in weight, wrinkles and lines in our skin, decline in sexual response, leaking bladders, forgetfulness, all seem a high price to pay for the freedom from menstruation and childbearing. HRT is useful, but cannot prevent all the exigencies of the ageing process. We do not bring it on ourselves. It simply happens. Is HRT the answer to all that happens around this time of life? The answer is an unequivocal NO. We have to accept the ageing process and the change in shape that this may bring. HRT may help the skin to remain firmer and it may help us to sleep so that bags under our eyes are less of a problem, but we need to accept the physical changes and learn to grow old with grace. At the same time, we can remain healthy and attractive through a good diet, exercise and enjoyment of life. There is no doubt that wrinkles are made worse by worry, and laughter has been shown to keep hearts healthy.

Perhaps we can echo Susan Sarandon's words, 'I look forward to being older, when what you look like becomes less and less an issue and what you are is the point.'

Summary

- In midlife it is impossible to escape the ageing process and 'the middle-age spread', or at least a change in body shape.
- HRT does not appear to contribute to weight gain, although lower doses of hormones can be helpful in reducing fluid retention and breast heaviness.
- As in other periods of life, a healthy diet and plenty of exercise will keep us looking good.
- Most important of all is enjoyment of life, combined with mental and spiritual growth.

16

Not waving, drowning –
dealing with depression

One does not discover new continents without consenting to lose sight of the shore for a very long time.

André Gide (1869–1951)

The menopause is a time of biological transition. It is a time when some women literally 'lose sight of the shore for a very long time', and it can also be a time of discovery. Women are understandably confused because some say that everything that happens around this time may be attributed to hormone deficiency, giving them hope of a quick fix, while others say that whatever is happening at this time is all in the mind, is nothing to do with hormones and that, in fact, hormone deficiency is a fiction. Nowhere is this thinking more confused than in the area of depression. Is depression *caused* by the menopause? If not, is it made worse by the hormone changes?

The menopausal woman has often been portrayed as depressed, anxious and low in self-esteem. But surveys of general populations, rather than menopause clinics, contradict the assertion that menopause has a negative effect on mental health. No increase in the incidence of *major* depression associated with natural menopause has been noted. Professor

Lorraine Dennerstein, reporting on the Melbourne Women's Midlife Health Project, says: 'Happiness appears to be enjoyed by the majority of Australian women in the midlife years; this contradicts negative stereotypes. Depression is related to poor health, stress, life events and negative attitude rather than to menopause.'

However, I have found in my own practice that hormone deficiency (both of estrogen or progesterone) results, in some women, in significant changes in mood and non-reproductive behaviour such as the ability to concentrate and even learn new facts, leading to fuzzy thinking and memory lapses. In general, estrogen excites and progesterone depresses mood. Women who have suffered from the mood swings that we call premenstrual syndrome, or PMS, have experienced this imbalance already. In this situation there may be too much estrogen and too little progesterone.

Menopause serves to exaggerate depressive tendencies already present, but psychosocial factors are the most common cause of distress at midlife and HRT is not a panacea for all of this, since hormone deficiency is not the major cause. Men suffer more frequently from substance abuse and hostility/conduct disorders at midlife, whereas women are more prone to develop anxiety disorders and depressive illness. In fact, women suffer more in this way than men – whether they are menopausal or not.

Estrogen therapy has been shown to reduce anxiety and *mild* depression in menopausal women. Women on HRT claim improvement in fine motor skills and memory. They are also less likely to develop dementing illness. Many more studies are needed in this area though before we can prescribe HRT solely to improve brain function, and given the recent negative reviews of HRT it is doubtful whether any woman would choose to use it to improve brain function alone unless sound evidence was found for this. The most recent study in the *New England Journal of Medicine* was released online on the Internet six weeks ahead of publication because it was considered to be of major importance. In this study of over 16,000 women, who were followed up for at least three years, it was declared that HRT does not improve the quality of life for women, suggesting that not only may it pose some risks for women taking it but it may have no benefits either. The women in the study were aged from 50 to 79. They did not have symptoms of hormone deficiency such as hot flushes or vaginal dryness, and they were given Premarin with a progestogen.

It is not really surprising that they did not have any measurable increase in quality of life since the main effect of HRT, especially the estrogen component, is to improve quality of life by relieving symptoms due to estrogen deficiency. I doubt that any physicians these days would put a woman on HRT for the rather vague reason of 'improvement in quality of life' in the absence of such symptoms.

In this chapter we will explore true depression, the woman who is 'not waving but drowning'. As in Stevie Smith's poem which talks about the man out at sea who 'was much too far out all his life' and 'not waving but drowning', many women are waving desperately, their plea for help misinterpreted as lighthearted social interaction, rather than a cry of distress, and therefore ignored.

A half century ago, it was common for women at midlife to be given barbiturates and very little sympathy if they appeared to be not coping with or withdrawing from life. Some of them were locked away in asylums; some locked themselves away in their own homes. Then Valium and Serepax became the popular antidepressants and many women were said to be 'hooked' on these. But the real problem was not addiction so much as failure to understand the process that was going on. *It is to be hoped that these days a correct diagnosis can be made of depression, which is not just temporary mood disturbance but possibly a life-threatening disorder.* HRT has a place in therapy, but it will not relieve longstanding true depression. *Women deserve to be heard. We must distinguish between waving and drowning.*

So what is depression? The best definition I know is 'the absence of joy'. It is a prolonged feeling of sadness plus the thought, 'I am worthless'. There may be other symptoms such as inability to sleep, decreased interest in sex and inability to work, but these are by no mean universal. There is often a sense of helplessness, a feeling of hopelessness and a lack of self-esteem.

I asked my own depressed patients to describe their feelings. Here are some of their descriptions:

'It's like living in a pool of pain; I'm helpless to escape from it.'
'I've fallen down a well; the sides are slippery. I can't get out.'
'I'm dragging down the whole family. They'd be better off without me.'
'It's painful to be with people. Life feels empty and meaningless.'
'Every minor obstacle feels like an impassable barrier.'
'I've failed. I'm worthless.'
'When I'm alone I stop believing that I exist.'

And Lydia gives a more detailed description below.

Lydia describes how she wakes each day with a sick empty feeling, a feeling of dread. How can she endure another day? Nothing interests her. Nothing tastes good. It is not worth getting up. She is aged 51. Her periods ceased a year ago. She was given HRT because of her hot flushes. She is sleeping better than she had been sleeping but still wakes early. She has been on antidepressants of different kinds for the last ten years. Her mother was always depressed. Lydia grew up in a household where nothing was ever discussed. Her mother used to retreat to bed – sometimes for days at a time.

Lydia's husband does not understand what is wrong with her. He works long hours and when at home watches TV and does not talk much. Lydia has lost interest in sex. They don't talk about this.

Lydia was pregnant when she got married. She had always wanted to have a career but she became a housewife and had three children in quick succession. After each child she had postnatal depression, though it was not called that. Her middle son has gone off the rails and has been on drugs and in prison. Her mother now has dementia and her father has had a stroke. They are still both in their own home and Lydia visits them every day. Lydia does not feel loved by anyone and she has no self-esteem at all. She feels trapped by life and her circumstances. She took an overdose of sleeping tablets last year and was given a lecture about this but no-one has ever helped her to look at what is happening. Lydia is drowning. I sent Lydia to a psychiatrist who is helping her to find a way to deal with her low self-esteem and her longstanding depression, which seems to be mirroring her mother's depression.

Some women I see do not know or believe that they are loved or even lovable. Many women are martyrs. They spend their whole lives living for others and never for themselves. A martyr has been described as 'life's sorriest victim', and this could be used to describe Rosina.

Rosina first saw me eight years ago. She had had a hysterectomy and one ovary removed at the age of 45. Hot flushes began soon after this. Over the next ten years various types of HRT were given, but she remained depressed and anxious and continued to have hot flushes. She said that she had had 'bad nerves' for years.

'I live my life for everyone else', she said. As she was growing up, her parents, especially her mother, told her 'how to be: how to talk, sit, dress, walk, even to laugh'.

Rosina was severely depressed and her estrogen levels were very low. I inserted an estrogen implant and sent her to see a psychiatrist. Over the next six months dramatic changes occurred. She says, now, that she feels she has her own life back rather than being the way other people want her to be. The implant gave her good levels of estrogens, settled her hot flushes and gave her more mental as well as physical energy, but the psychotherapy turned everything around for her psychologically. She was given a mild antidepressant but she had been given this before without much improvement, so I do not believe that this was the reason for her dramatic improvement. The real key to her recovery was that she was willing to explore all the negative messages and feelings that had kept her from feeling, tasting and enjoying life.

Rosina had a deprived upbringing. She was born in Italy, the second child of a farm labourer. Her father migrated to Australia when she was four years old and her mother was left to work to support the family. As a result of this, she feels that she lost her childhood. She was sexually abused by the uncle who lived with them, but her poor relationship with her mother left her unable to explain the difficulties she was encountering. The family came to Australia when she was fifteen so her parents were reunited after eleven years; it is not surprising that the family was dysfunctional. Her mother had two more children and was more nurturing of these than of the two born in Italy. Her supportive older brother died at age 50 and she could not mourn him despite her sense of enormous loss. Her mother lives on the farm and never contacts Rosina.

After Rosina regained some emotional balance, she contacted her mother and has since continued to do this, but her mother remains cold and distant. By coming to terms with 'who she is', Rosina is now happy and the depression has lifted. She says, 'Now I have the strength to be myself, to be exactly what I want to be and where I want to be.' She has a loving and supportive husband and children who have always been there for her, but until she found her lost self even their love could not keep her from depression and low self-esteem. Nor can HRT alone relieve deep depression, the result of abandonment first by others, and then by self. On at least one occasion Rosina had considered suicide.

Why do some women suicide at this time? Self-loathing is all too often the reason. It has been said that people commit suicide for only one reason – to escape torment.

'We cannot blot out one page of our lives', said the novelist George Sand, 'but we can throw the book in the fire.' Virginia Woolf, who wrote with such feeling about the necessity for a woman to have 'a room of one's own', achieved this herself so that she had the freedom to write. She would become one of our greatest writers, but could not cope with her untreated depression and, at the age of 59, she drowned herself.

The message of this chapter is that depression at midlife is not primarily caused by the hormone deficiencies of the menopause. HRT will help to lift mood in those who were not previously depressed, but is not appropriate as the only treatment for severe depression. The latter needs full investigation and appropriate psychological help and medication. Feelings of loss and grief at this stage of life may aggravate previously dormant depression. Giving a woman space and time to talk about her feelings and her fears is of major importance. Those who cannot talk to anyone, or who talk but feel unheard, are most likely to withdraw from life. Some commit suicide. Some simply retreat and can no longer connect with anyone, least of all themselves.

Those who cannot talk to anyone, or who talk but feel unheard, are most likely to withdraw from life. Some commit suicide.

As always, Shakespeare says it so well:

Give sorrow words: the grief that does not speak
Whispers the o'er-fraught heart and bids it break.

Macbeth 5.1.50-1

Not depressed, just lonely

The mass of men lead lives of quiet desperation.

Henry David Thoreau (1817–1862)

It is sadly true that many people, and particularly women, live lives of quiet desperation and also isolation. Guiseppina is such a woman.

Guiseppina is now aged 55. She is a beautiful woman with smooth, unwrinkled skin, remarkably well preserved for our hot, dry climate. Her doctor referred her, asking me to 'treat her depression'. He thought she might need hormones and possibly antidepressants as well. Her menopause occurred two years ago. She had some flooding for six months before her periods ceased. Since then she has had a few flushes. She says she feels hot much of the time without much episodic flushing. She is sleeping quite well, but when she wakes each morning it is with some gloom. She wonders 'What am I here for? What am I supposed to do today?'

She says, 'I don't think I am important to anyone. I have become superfluous.' She acknowledges that she is a good housewife and a good cook, but even these attributes do not seem, to her, to be worthwhile. She feels largely unappreciated. Her two children are married. Her daughter has two children and works part-time. Her husband Gino is 60 and had to retire two years ago with a bad back caused by work. He spends much of his day with his male cronies at the Italian Club, playing cards and indoor bowls. Guiseppina is not really interested, nor has she ever been included, in these pursuits. She feels that Gino has deserted her when she most needs his company and support. She feels very tired, both emotionally and physically.

Gino and Guiseppina were born and grew up in a village in the south of Italy. Gino came to Australia as an eighteen-year-old and found a job as a farm labourer.

When he went back to Italy to visit his family five years later he met Guiseppina again. Their families arranged a marriage between them. They returned to Australia to an isolated country town. Guiseppina was then eighteen and could not speak English.

Gino worked hard and gradually got better jobs and they moved nearer to the city. Guiseppina involved herself in the care of her two children and gradually learned English with their help, but still does not read or write easily in her second language. Gino manages all the family business and finances.

Their daughter is very self-sufficient and ambitious. She has a good marriage. She does not think of herself as Italian though she speaks the language well. She has no real interest in meeting her parents' families in Italy. She rarely asks her mother to babysit, and since she is not often home on weekdays and is busy at weekends with her own family, Guiseppina feels left out and useless.

Guiseppina has no interest in sex, which she knows is partly because she resents Gino for abandoning her, and there is very little joy in her life. Earlier depression was described as 'the absence of joy', but I don't think she is clinically depressed. In fact she agreed with my diagnosis, that she is *not depressed, just lonely*. She attends her church (without Gino) but has not made any real friends there. Her mother, now aged 83 and frail, still lives in the same village in which she was born. Her two brothers and one sister are still living close to their birthplace. She has only been back there once, when her father died. She no longer feels part of this close family.

Guiseppina has tried to talk to Gino about her feelings, her sadness, and her sense of not belonging, of no longer having a role in life. He cannot understand why she is lonely. He is angry with her for no longer being interested in sex. The doctor who sent her to me had already started her on a small dose of antidepressants, but it was too early to tell if this had been helpful. A blood test had showed that she had a low iron count. This was a result of her heavy bleeding just before menopause. She had also begun a course of iron tablets, which would help with the tiredness. Her thyroid function was normal so this was not a reason for her tiredness.

I didn't believe that HRT or the antidepressants would be of much use, so I just allowed her to talk about all her feelings of desertion and worthlessness. A month later she felt much better about herself. She said that being listened to sympathetically had been helpful. I put her in touch with a charity group who needed volunteers. She had already met two women in this group who had also been lonely and had found a way to deal with it.

So for Guiseppina it was not her hormones causing her distress but feelings of social isolation for which she was not directly responsible.

This is not a rare story. There is social isolation nowadays that was almost unknown a century ago. In a *Time* cover story Robert Wright discussed the issues that cause sadness to become debilitating depression, and anxiety to become chronic and paralysing. Social isolation is a major cause, and the life of some housewives in suburbia is a classic example. Women like Guiseppina who have migrated halfway across the world, have been detached from home and family, and have been totally dependent in every way on a man who now has little time for them long to be heard and seen and valued. In the 1950s such women were given barbiturates to dull their emotional pain. Many of them retreated into their homes and a few of them developed agoraphobia.

> There is social isolation nowadays that was almost unknown a century ago ... [causing] sadness to become debilitating depression, and anxiety to become chronic and paralysing.

Modern antidepressants and HRT are also not the answer to deep sadness and loneliness. So what or who can help? A compassionate doctor who takes the time to listen and then refers these women on to some kind of support system is what is required.

Summary

- Women during midlife may suffer true depression, but this is generally not related to hormone deficiency; rather, psycho-social factors are usually the cause. However, feelings of loss and grief at menopause may amplify existing depressive tendencies.
- Seeking help for severe depression is enormously important because it is not simply mood disturbance, and can be life threatening.
- Estrogen therapy may reduce anxiety and mild depression in menopausal women, but does not appear to improve quality of life.
- Many women experience feelings of isolation, worthlessness and deep sadness during menopause. Enabling women to talk about their feelings and experiences and encouraging them to seek support is essential for their wellbeing.

17

Sticks and stones *may* break my bones –
preventing osteoporosis

The cure for this ill is not to sit still
Or frowst with a book by the fire
But to take a large hoe and a shovel also
And dig till you gently perspire.

Rudyard Kipling (1865–1936)

Physical activity is a vital component of a healthy lifestyle and essential for disease prevention. The average woman will live at least 25 years beyond menopause and, during these years, regular physical activity can improve her quality of life, her general health and sense of wellbeing.

Even at menopause, fitness can reduce the risk of heart disease, osteoporosis and diabetes, yet only 38 percent of women over 19 exercise regularly. Exercise should be encouraged and prescribed.

My interest in the menopause began in 1978 when Professor Christopher Nordin came as a visiting professor to the university department in which I was working. He challenged me to consider the effects of the menopause on the whole woman, not just their bones. He is a recognised expert in the field of osteoporosis but he takes the wider view and has done major research. I acknowledge my debt to him.

Osteoporosis, the so-called 'silent epidemic', is feared by the elderly. A study reported in the *British Medical Journal* showed that many older women 'would rather be dead than experience the loss of independence and quality of life that results from a bad hip fracture and admission to a nursing home. Any loss of ability to live independently in the community has a considerable detrimental effect on their quality of life.' Women want to know how they can prevent osteoporosis.

At 80 Elsie was very fit for her age. She could walk 5 to 10 kilometres per day and went swimming in the ocean. She looked after a large garden. She was thin and agile. Her mind was still sharp: she taught adult literacy classes and ran a poetry circle. She had never married. She was a career schoolteacher in the days when such women remained single. She was my English teacher in my matriculation years and the person of greatest influence in my life. Soon after her 80th birthday she stepped on the garden hose and twisted her leg. She did not fall directly onto her hip but nevertheless it broke. Her life changed utterly. She was never able to walk properly from that time and was, until her death at 99, confined to bed or a wheelchair. She had to go into a nursing home.

At her retirement she had planned to live in her own home, with paid help, when she got older. She had looked after her own parents in their own home until they died. Her quality of life was drastically reduced and she had to rely on others for most of her needs. If she had not had osteoporosis, I think that she would have remained physically active and relatively independent for her whole life.

If Elsie's bone density had been measured in her sixties or even her seventies, her osteoporosis could have been treated and fracture prevented. *It is never too late to take preventive measures.* Despite all the exercise she did, there were other factors causing bone loss. She had never taken much calcium in her diet, and of course she went through menopause before the days of HRT, so her bone density was never measured.

Osteoporosis may be related to menopause but is not purely caused by it. The major factor at menopause is the loss of our hormones, particularly estrogen.

When periods cease for longer than six months (at any age), estrogen levels plummet and there is an accelerated loss of calcium from the bones. This occurs, for instance, in young women who starve themselves to the point where their periods stop. The calcium pulled out of the bones is lost in the urine; this known as 'obligatory loss'. Blood calcium levels must be kept steady at all times as calcium is so important in cellular function, so if calcium is pulled out of bone and can't get back (in the absence of estrogens) it will pass out in the urine. When women take estrogens this obligatory loss is prevented.

Incidentally, measuring calcium levels in the blood is *not* a way to diagnose osteoporosis or to find out if there is adequate calcium in the diet. Measuring calcium levels in the urine will show if there is excessive loss. Very high blood levels of calcium in the blood may indicate disease of the parathyroid glands or some types of cancer, but low levels are not diagnostic of osteoporosis. The level of calcium in the blood is kept constant unless there is disease of the kinds mentioned above. The effect of the loss of calcium from the bones depends on the bone density achieved prior to menopause, the 'peak bone mass', which we have by the age of 35. This depends on factors such as our genes, exercise, and calcium in the diet. Women at menopause may feel tired and lack motivation to exercise, so may exercise less just when they need to do more. Also at this time, there may be other disorders affecting glands such as the thyroid and parathyroid, which will cause loss of bone density.

Lifestyle factors, such as smoking and drinking more than moderate amounts of alcohol, may also affect bone density. Some medications, notably cortisone and derivatives, taken orally for several months, will cause osteoporosis. The bone depletion caused by loss of hormones lasts for several years and can be reversed by taking HRT.

Osteoporosis is a measurable condition. It is not always predictable from medical history or family history. We know that there is a genetic link, so choosing one's parents would help if this were possible. Sometimes there is a distinct family history which alerts us – mother and grandmother may have shrunk as they grew older or may have had a fracture with 'minimal trauma', such as tripping on sticks or stones.

What do we mean by minimal trauma? Elsie had such a fracture. She did not fall heavily but merely tripped on a garden hose. I have heard of strapping grandsons hugging a grandmother and fracturing one or more of her ribs.

I believe it is useful to measure bone density in all women at menopause. Others believe that is not necessary if a woman is taking hormones anyway, but will then measure bone density after HRT has ceased.

The results of a study in Australia ... indicate that 60 percent of women and 30 percent of men suffer from an osteoporotic fracture after the age of 60 years.

Measurement of bone density is best done on DEXA machines which use very low dose X-rays. The X-rays do not go right through bone as with normal X-rays but are reflected back into the machine in varying amounts, depending on the density of the bone. This is called reflective absorptiometry. The hip and the lumbar spine are the sites usually measured. Ultrasound techniques were used on the forearm before the DEXA machines became available and are still useful in research.

Osteoporosis is potentially preventable. We can change our lifestyle. HRT is still the gold standard treatment to prevent bone loss due to hormone deficiency, though recent studies suggest that long-term HRT may have risks that outweigh the benefit for bones. Other medications are being developed which act on bones only. Estrogen 'look-alikes', such as raloxifen, are available. They are called SERMs (selective estrogen receptor modulators). These act like estrogens in bones to stop further loss, but they do not stop (and may even increase) hot flushes and vaginal dryness. They do not stimulate breast tissue, so the risk of breast cancer may even be decreased for some women. The best-known SERM is tamoxifen, which is already being used for breast cancer prevention or treatment.

Osteoporosis affects men as well as women, though men do not have the accelerated loss due to menopause and at all ages they have higher bone density than women. The results of a study in Australia – the Dubbo Osteoporosis Epidemiology Study (DOES) – indicate that 60 percent of women and 30 percent of men suffer from an osteoporotic fracture after the age of 60 years. In this study 10 percent of fractures in 60–79-year-olds were hip fractures, compared to 40 percent in the group aged 80 or more.

Hip fracture is associated with a death rate of 20 percent in the first twelve months, and 25 percent (like Elsie) remain in nursing homes for the rest of their lives. No wonder that the elderly fear osteoporosis.

Prevention of osteoporosis is a major public health concern. At present there are no medications capable of *fully* restoring lost bone density to the depleted skeleton. Is it possible to maintain bone density without HRT? Yes, but it is not easy. Lifestyle factors are very important. Women at midlife need to ensure good calcium intake, as supplements, if not in the diet; 1200 to 1500 milligrams daily is recommended. Physical activity such as walking for 45 minutes briskly three times a week can help to prevent further loss. Weight-bearing exercise, resistance training and high-intensity fitness regimes can reduce fracture risk, but the latter regimes are not suitable for the frail elderly and may increase the risk of falls. A two-year study, which my colleague, Professor Richard Prince, and I conducted fifteen years ago (reported in the *New England Journal of Medicine,* October 1991), showed that exercise, calcium supplementation and HRT were all useful in preventing further decrease in bone density, but HRT was the most effective, and the combination of all three was obviously desirable in some women.

Having thin bones is only one side of the story. Fractures are usually caused by falls (or coughing or bear hugs, as mentioned above), so we must prevent falls in the elderly. Balance is vital. Both exercise and HRT may help to improve this. Women who go through menopause with few symptoms are usually reluctant to take HRT. Some women, even though symptomatic, refuse to take HRT because of the perceived risk of breast cancer.

Mavis, aged 61, came to see me recently. At the age of 51 she went through menopause. Although she had hot flushes and other symptoms, she was reluctant to take HRT because of her fear of breast cancer. Her mother had breast cancer, but died at 85 after fracturing her hip. Mavis had very low bone density in both hip and spine. HRT was recommended, but she preferred to take calcium and some herbal remedies.

She reported to her doctor with backache. Bone density was now well below the fracture line. I sent her for an X-ray of her upper spine. This revealed early fractures in two vertebrae. These are called wedge fractures because they shorten the front edge of the vertebra and will eventually cause the bend in the spine called the dowager's hump.

It was a pity that preventive measures were not taken, but it is not too late to prevent further fractures and deformity. Mavis is taking a drug called alendronate (Fosamax), which will improve bone density. It is an expensive drug, but the Australian health system provides it more cheaply because Mavis had already had a fracture with minimal trauma; in her case there was no actual trauma as the vertebra broke under the weight of the spinal column. It is considered that once a fracture with minimal trauma has occurred the risk of further such fractures is increased.

Thus, in one sense, it is never too late to treat osteoporosis, but prevention is better than cure. The question, 'Is it me or my hormones', is a vital one in the area of osteoporosis. The answer is that it is usually both.

Summary

- Osteoporosis is a condition feared by the elderly, so it is essential that bone density be measured at menopause.
- Osteoporosis is preventable. HRT certainly prevents bone loss due to hormone deficiency, but long-term use may have other risks. Other medications are also becoming available.
- Lifestyle factors are also very important in prevention – good calcium intake, physical activity, drinking only in moderation and not smoking.
- A new drug is now available which can improve bone density. It is very expensive but is provided more cheaply in Australia to those who have experienced a fracture with minimal trauma.

18

Staying abreast of things –
cancer risk in midlife

The day is gone and all its sweets are gone
Sweet voice, sweet lips, soft hand and softer breasts.

Keats (1795–1821)

The Romantic poets and artists have long waxed lyrical over breasts – to them the sign of woman's beauty as well as motherhood. *The Oxford Dictionary* cites the breasts as the 'source of nourishment', but also says that they are 'heart, emotions and thoughts'. No wonder that a woman's breasts are very important to her and usually to her sexual partner as well.

In the last 30 years the true function of the female breast has been rediscovered and breastfeeding has regained its rightful place as the most appropriate way to nurture the newborn.

Many women choose to fully breastfeed for at least one year and some continue for two years. My colleague, Professor Peter Hartman, head of Biochemistry at the University of Western Australia, is a leading researcher in the field of lactation and I was privileged to be involved in some of his research into factors that affect breastfeeding in our modern society.

In my time in New Guinea, I saw that most women fully breastfed their babies for two years and then partly breastfed for another year. We had to deter village women from using a bottle with artificial milk since they had no means of sterilisation or properly measuring formula. It was amazing to see older women (grandmothers) with shrunken breasts able to start lactating again and feeding orphaned babies.

So it is not the size, shape or age of breasts that determines function. Bigger is not necessarily better, though regarded by some as more beautiful or more sexually arousing. Thus breasts have a very important role to play in society. In primitive society the breasts are valued for their function, whereas in modern society they have become sex objects (e.g. Julia Roberts used hers to great advantage in the film, *Erin Brockovich* – 'Boobs, Ed' she tells her partner who can't see how she has managed to extract information from certain men). Dolly Parton, Marilyn Monroe, Jane Russell and many others also achieved mammary fame.

Breasts can be painful and even unsightly, yet most women fear to lose a breast to cancer because, as one of my women patients confided to me, 'It is hard to hide the removal of a breast.'

Sara had cervical cancer in her thirties resulting in a hysterectomy, but she shrugged this off saying, 'Well, who can tell?' However, in her fifties the discovery of a suspicious lump in her breast and the possibility of a mastectomy filled her with dread and shame. 'I regarded the lump in my breast as more frightening than the cervical cancer. I coped with that well; it was an "inside" job. I could hide it. But if you lose a breast everybody is going to know your secret.' She described the process of diagnosis in a breast clinic at a large hospital: 'There were many of us all being processed. The staff members were considerate and kind, but in another sense we were just numbers and it might not even have been cancer for some. In the first room, we sat upright in our chairs and chatted a bit to each other. In the next room, most of us slumped down and were silent as we waited for biopsy results. In the third room women were openly weeping, some inconsolably. There was an atmosphere of gloom. My results were good. I had a benign lesion. I left the room smiling, relieved and reprieved but still somewhat shaken at my escape.'

That HRT may cause breast cancer is the main reason why many women refuse to use it even though other therapies are less effective in relieving menopausal symptoms. So the familiar question arises when a woman develops breast cancer, 'Was it me or my hormones?' Or perhaps: 'Was it me or the hormones I was given?'

Jane is a feisty woman who works as a school nurse at a large private boys' school. This involves long hours and considerable responsibility, although she says that the rewards are worth it (not least the fund of stories that she collects from the boys and passes on to me at each visit!). She had a hysterectomy years ago for heavy bleeding; one ovary was left in but did not function well thereafter, so she began HRT. Various tablets and the patch were tried but she seemed to need more estrogen than these gave, so I inserted an estrogen implant. We found that a dose of 50 mg of estradiol lasted her about six months. She had breasts that were quite active and became sore when the implants were first inserted, but they were not unduly uncomfortable and she was not concerned about this. I had explained to her that estrogens stimulate breast tissue and can increase activity in the breasts but that I did not believe that they caused breast cancer, though a lesion already present could be stimulated to grow. She accepted this and asked to continue with implants because she felt so well physically and mentally. Working with boys, she needed all her wits about her and felt embarrassed if she had hot flushes, got flustered or lost things. She had regular mammograms, which reported that her breasts were dense; this was consistent with estrogen stimulation.

She had been on HRT for six years when she found a breast lump, which proved to be malignant on biopsy. She had a partial mastectomy. Her lymph glands were clear. She was told not to have any further estrogen therapy. Her surgeon prescribed tamoxifen, which is an anti-estrogen used to prevent recurrence of breast cancer and is also used as a preventive measure in women with a close relative with breast cancer. Her hot flushes returned with a vengeance. Her breast tissue at the site of surgery became infected and the resultant scar has remained painful and angry. After a year she elected to go back on low-dose estrogen therapy, having tried alternatives without obtaining any relief of symptoms. This year she has started on tibolone, the non-estrogen containing HRT, with good relief of symptoms.

Marian, aged 53, came to see me as she was having hot flushes and sleeplessness and altogether felt miserable. Her mother had developed breast cancer at 75, but was still alive. Marian was terrified of developing breast cancer herself. I told her that I believed that taking HRT would not alter her chances, and would certainly relieve her symptoms, but she remained unconvinced. She was also concerned about the dangers of mammograms, as she had been told by 'someone who knew' that these may cause cancer. I explained that I had no other remedies to offer her because she was having classic estrogen deficiency symptoms, which would best respond to estrogens. I urged her to have a mammogram, but she said she would have to think about it. She went away rather sorrowful. A year later she rang me to say that she had finally decided to have a mammogram, which had detected a very early cancer. It was small, so she had a lumpectomy only. Her glands were not affected so she did not have to have radiotherapy.

I must confess that I was rather relieved. If I had persuaded her to take HRT it would certainly have been blamed for the cancer!

There is no doubt that estrogen therapy will make a sensitive cancer grow. Such a tumour is described as estrogen-receptor positive. Pathologists check breast cancers for estrogen receptors. If these are present, it suggests that estrogens have probably accelerated the growth of the cancer since cells are able to take up estrogen and use it as a growth factor. Most breast surgeons forbid patients to have any estrogen therapy after this. I can remember some 40 years ago when surgeons pursued every last bit of estrogen in the body by taking out ovaries, the adrenal glands and finally the pituitary gland. This was barbaric surgery indeed and, although it occasionally prolonged life, it was at the expense of any quality of life. Fortunately this terrorist warfare on women's bodies has been abandoned.

The genetic risk of cancer, where women carry a specific gene, is only about 5 percent of all breast cancers. BRCA1 and BRCA2 are the genes so far identified. The family history of these unfortunate women is definite and daunting. At least half of the breast cancers have no estrogen receptors, so it is not primarily to do with hormone stimulation but rather to a change in the genes in the cells that leads to breast cancer — usually at a young age. In the USA, with its large population compared to Australia's, there are many such families and many young women have both breasts removed before the age of 40 as a preventive measure.

Sian was aged 48 when she called me at home just before Christmas one year. I had delivered her only child eight years before. She was premenopausal and was having heavy periods, but she was most concerned about her lumpy painful breasts. She was frightened and quite convinced that she had cancer. A mammogram was not easy to read because of the breast density. An ultrasound showed many cysts. A surgeon performed multiple biopsies and she was found to have many very active areas. On the biopsy of one of these there was an early cancer. She had a mastectomy. The glands were clear, fortunately. Within a year the other breast was found to have some suspicious areas.

She elected to have this breast removed also. Pathology showed widespread precancerous change.

There is no doubt that Sian's own estrogen hormones had been causing the overactivity of her breast glands and encouraging the growth of the abnormal cells. Sian has always been a worrier. She has brought up her only child alone when her marriage failed. She had this baby when she was 40 and was not able to breastfeed. These factors — stress, late first baby, and lack of breastfeeding — are thought to be risk factors for breast cancer. Another risk factor which has been cited is diet. High fat in the diet was thought to be a factor, but this has not been substantiated in recent studies; however, more than one standard drink of alcohol daily has been shown to increase breast cancer risk by altering the excretion of estrogens by the liver.

The death rate from breast cancer is decreasing because many cancers are now picked up at an early stage.

Is the incidence of breast cancer increasing? Yes, because more cases are being picked up as the result of good breast cancer screening. The death rate from breast cancer is decreasing because many cancers are now picked up at an early stage. Women are more likely to die in their sixties and seventies from heart attack and stroke than from breast cancer, but breast cancer strikes at what, in our society, is so valued by women (and their partners also) and thus it is tremendously emotive.

Estrogens are not to be feared, but they should certainly be treated with great respect. Estrogen therapy must be used with care and caution. If breasts overreact to the therapy being given, then that therapy must be stopped or the dose reduced. As we have seen, however, tibolone is an alternative that many specialists believe can be used to relieve estrogen deficiency symptoms without stimulating the breast tissue. The SERMs, tamoxifen and raloxifen, as mentioned previously, have an anti-estrogen effect in the breast so are used in women who have had breast cancer or have an increased risk of breast cancer. They do not suppress hot flushes and may even make them worse.

As discussed earlier in the book, direct causation of breast cancer by estrogens has never been proven. However, estrogens certainly promote the growth and division of breast tissue. This is their job in the reproductive years as the body is prepared each month for possible pregnancy. After menopause, when estrogen production by the ovaries ceases, the incidence of breast cancer starts to rise whether a woman takes estrogen therapy or not. This increase is at least partly due to the effect of ageing on the cells.

It has been scientifically proven that the human papilloma virus (HPV) causes one type of cervical cancer. And there are carcinogens (cancer-producing agents) in tobacco smoke which may cause lung cancer.

A study done ten years ago on a group of women aged 80 and over who had died of causes other than breast cancer showed that 25 percent of these women, at autopsy, had a previously undiagnosed breast cancer. In some cases the cancer was visible and had been kept hidden by the woman. The breast cancer was an incidental finding; the major cause of death in these women was heart attack or stroke.

The study thus suggests that breast cancers may grow slowly. Giving HRT to a woman with an existent breast cancer may make it grow faster. This is the message that we need to act on. So the answer to the question: 'Is it me or my hormones that has caused the breast cancer'? is 'It is probably neither'. However, diet and stress factors may have contributed to the cancer. Estrogens are activators of breast lesions, both benign and malignant, so must be used with care and perhaps avoided altogether in some women. Certainly a woman who has had a breast cancer with positive estrogen receptors would be told not to take HRT after this event, even though studies done by Wren and Eden and their group in Sydney have shown that giving HRT to such women did not increase the risk of cancer recurrence over that of a group who did not take HRT.

Summary

- In primitive societies the breasts are valued for their true function, while in Western society they are often seen as sex objects.
- It is for this reason that women find it harder to accept that they have breast cancer than any other cancer and why it receives so much media attention.
- The genetic risk of breast cancer is quite low.
- Factors such as stress, late first baby, lack of breastfeeding and excessive consumption of alcohol appear to increase breast cancer risk.
- The incidence of breast cancer rises after menopause whether a woman has estrogen therapy or not, but the major cause of death of women in their sixties and seventies is heart attack or stroke.
- Direct causation of breast cancer by estrogens has not been proven; however, giving HRT to women with an existing breast cancer may cause it to grow faster.
- Estrogen therapy must be used with care and caution.

Part 3

Sexuality and relationship

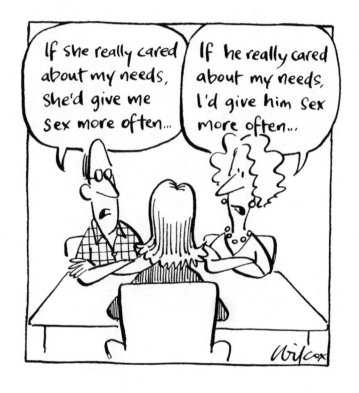

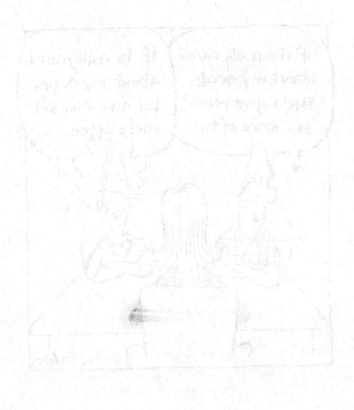

19

Midlife sexuality –
I'm too hot and he snores!

Menopausal changes cause a progressive loss of libido and a crisis of the self-perception as an object of desire.

Dr Alessandra Graziottin, Director, Center of Gynecology and
Medical Sexology, Milan, Italy

Sexuality, at any age, was little discussed in my medical training. With the introduction of the oral contraceptive pill in the 1960s came a new freedom for women, and sexuality was more openly discussed. But decline in sexual function at midlife for women was still largely ignored and women suffered in silence. It was well known that many men sought younger women as their wife's interest in sex faded. For women there may be multiple problems causing a decline in libido and there is unlikely to be a magic cure which fixes them all. Nothing analogous to Viagra for men!

Stress may be a factor and stress has many facets, such as family and work problems, change in image, loss of energy and sleeplessness. And, yes, as the title of this chapter suggests, 'I'm too hot and he snores', so partners may have to resort to sleeping in separate beds or in different rooms. This for her is a relief, but he may be less willing to go and get

162 IS IT ME OR MY HORMONES?

help for his snoring than she is to get help for her flushes and reduced libido. The relationship may have become so comfortable as to be totally bland.

No excitement, routine boring positions. Romance has given way to duty and boredom.

There are some physical barriers in the woman which can be removed. Lack of feeling, interest and response in the woman may be related to hormonal deficiencies, but usually has a psychological basis as well. One woman put it in a nutshell: 'It's the time of life. I'm emotionally cold and physically hot.' If a woman's lifestyle is frenetic, this may act as an anti-aphrodisiac as well. Women comparing their stories with each other will find many striking similarities.

It is common to find a waning of sexual interest as sex hormone levels decrease, but it is rarely hormone levels, alone, which cause this.

As discussed in Michelle's story in Chapter 7, 'It can't be menopause – you're too young', replacement therapy may need to include testosterone as well as estrogen. However, libido is not merely balanced hormones; it is also about balance in your relationship.

Dr Alessandra Graziottin, a gynaecologist who has done much valuable research into sexual dysfunction, particularly at midlife, has this to say:

Libido is a comprehensive yet elusive term, a Latin word that means desire. It was first used by Sigmund Freud to indicate the energy corresponding to the psychic side of the sex drive. Carl Jung defined libido in a wider sense, as the psychic energy in all that is 'appetitus' a kind of 'desire towards', not necessarily sexual.

The subjective experience of sex is accompanied by, and partly consists of, various physiological changes, many of which are preparations for sexual behaviour.

Psychological processes play an important role in human libido; we learn to feel sexual drive at certain times and in certain situations.

In recent years the realm of the libido has grown to include a deeper understanding of its biological roots and of its vulnerability to personal factors and external agents.

Dr Graziottin goes on to explain the difference between sexual arousal and sexual desire, arousal being in the genitals and desire being a mental state, an attitude:

The brain is the very first sex organ as it is the biological and emotional realm of the libido. It is the brain that associates sensory stimuli and emotions ...; anticipates the pleasures of love; colours our erotic and emotional life with fantasies, dreams, erotic phantasms, sexual daydreams ...

For many women I see, these two states are confused and they, and their partners, expect that hormones will fix everything.

Hormones do affect sexual function in women. Estrogens are necessary to keep tissues healthy and responsive, particularly the vaginal lining, which dries out without estrogens. They also seem to have an effect on the brain's ability to associate sensory stimuli and emotions. Testosterone also plays a part in libido and sexual desire.

> The brain is ... the very first sex organ, as it is the biological and emotional realm of the libido. It is the brain that ... anticipates the pleasures of love ...

Much more research is needed to better understand the biological basis of human libido, but hormone therapy has an important role in preserving sexual function.

Germaine Greer, in *The Whole Woman* (which I think is required reading for women at midlife just as *The Female Eunuch* was for the feminists in their young adulthood), has a chapter on sex. She says:

'Those of us who have experienced the waning of desire as a liberation are beyond redemption.' She is saying that for some women, and for some men also, lack of sexual activity is not a problem. Leave us alone. There does not need to be a standard to aspire to. But, for most people, for a relationship to remain alive, individual sexual needs *are* important and *do* need to be addressed. At this time of life the differences between the sexes are very obvious. *She* may suffer in silence; *he* may complain if she is not responsive and may seek sex elsewhere.

Germaine Greer also says, 'In sex, as in everything else, we imposed a performance ethic.' This idea of a performance ethic is well worth exploring. I see many women who feel that their sexual performance is not up to expectations. But whose expectations? Not just their husband's, it turns out, but those that seem to be 'the norm' for couples from a reading of various women's magazines. Thus it all becomes too much. What makes *me* happy? What makes *him* happy? What does *he* want? What do *I* want?

However, what we are talking about is a relationship issue not a competition.

Patricia and I have given many seminars together on 'brain sex' and this could almost be a book in itself. Men also have sexual problems but it is hard for them to acknowledge them or to seek help. *There are many women whose husbands are no longer able to satisfy them, but this side of things seems to be a conspiracy of silence.* I will tell Rosa's story to illustrate this.

Rosa is 52. She is a bountiful woman; very juicy is how I would best describe her. She has been married to George for 30 years and has three grown-up children. Her periods ceased at age 51 and she has had few flushes but is not sleeping very well. Her doctor prescribed HRT, which has settled the flushes but not the sleeping problem. She was somewhat embarrassed to tell me her real problem and in fact had not discussed this with her male doctor. *She* still feels very sexual, but

George seems to have switched off. He keeps making excuses for not having sex. Not just headaches! He stays up very late watching television and then sneaks into bed when he thinks she is asleep. Sometimes he sleeps in another room.

This is an unusual story. Many of my female patients say that they are the ones who stay up late and only go to bed when their husband is asleep. Rosa is very distressed. George refuses to discuss the matter and certainly does not think it is a problem. She asked him to go to their doctor or another doctor but he will not listen. A friend to whom she timidly confided the problem said that she was lucky; she wished that her own husband would be less sexually demanding! The other advice was to use a vibrator or find another partner.

I offered to talk to George but, not surprisingly, he did not take up this offer.

Three months later, and rather to my surprise, he phoned me. Rosa had threatened to leave him if he was not interested in sharing his problem and seeking help. He couldn't believe that she would just walk out. I sent him to see a specialist who found that his anti-hypertensive medication was causing some of his dysfunction. A change of medication helped, but the real breakthrough came when he agreed to go with Rosa to Patricia and her husband for relationship counselling.

Rosa did not just want sex; she was looking for sharing and intimacy.

Relationship issues must be clearly defined before hormone or any other therapy is given to solve sexual problems. 'Women want love and men want sex' seems a rather terse and simplistic summing up of the difference between the sexes, but it is basically true. Women, in my experience, mourn their loss of sexual response and also mourn their husbands' reaction to it. Many seek help for their husbands' sake rather than their own. They feel so guilty and, in fact, are sometimes made to feel guilty. They feel blamed, as if they have deliberately turned away, when in fact the fire has simply gone out. Love would help to reignite it but this is most often not offered, only criticism, which extinguishes the last low flame. Left alone, many would retire from the sexual scene. They would rather read a book and go to sleep than have the sexual gymnastics that are required of them. But this is simply not allowed or tolerated in many relationships, hence Germaine Greer's comment: 'Those of us who have experienced the waning of desire as liberation are beyond redemption.'

There are hormonal causes, in women, for sexual disinterest and dysfunction. What also needs to be explored – and it is beyond the scope of this book to do this – is the man's loss of interest. Erectile function is now treatable with Viagra, which replaces the less inviting methods such as local injections. It is well known that certain medical conditions such as hypertension and diabetes and the medications used to treat them may be a cause of impotence. But less willingly admitted to, or explored, are the emotional and psychological issues which men seem to prefer to sweep under the carpet, leaving wives such as Rosa to suffer in silence.

'Is it me or my hormones?' Rosa asked me. My reply was: 'It is neither. It is your husband who needs help!'

In the next chapter Patricia explores relationship issues and sexual expectations and differences, and gives guidance in the vital area of sexual relationship. As a doctor I was taught to be a fixer, a repairer of bodily functions, using hormone and other replacement therapy. I was taught very little about emotional issues. We learnt about the heart as a mechanical organ. The soul was never discussed. But the answer to the question 'Is it me or my hormones?' is 'It is you *and* your hormones.' Both can be helped. I will discuss some of the practicalities of hormone therapy, particularly the use of male hormone therapy (testosterone) for sexual problems in Chapter 21.

Summary

- Lack of libido in midlife is often caused by many factors: hormonal, relationship, stress, change in self-image, loss of energy, sleeplessness.
- Decrease in sex hormone levels will have an impact on a woman's sexual interest, but this is rarely the single cause.
- The brain is the main sex organ as it is the seat of both the biological and emotional components of the libido.
- For some women and men, lack of sexual activity is inconsequential; but for most a healthy sex life is important for a healthy relationship.
- Men need also to recognise if they have a sexual problem and to acknowledge any emotional or psychological issues, and to get help with them, particularly if their partner's wellbeing and the relationship are at risk because of these issues.
- Before hormone or other replacement therapy is given to women to solve sexual problems, it is crucial that relationship issues be defined and explored.

20

Sexuality and your relationship –
in need of the beloved

When you realise there is nothing lacking, the whole world belongs to you.

Lao Tzu (c. 604–531 BC)

For a woman, sexuality is very closely linked to relationship and at midlife they are almost impossible to separate. Sexuality for a woman is intrinsically linked to her relationship with her partner, her feelings of self-worth and her soul. There is no point trying to have a relationship with someone on the outside if you have lost, or never had, an intimate connection with yourself.

The unhealed wounds of love often present themselves in our sexual relationships at this time in our lives. When the question, 'Will we make love or won't we?', keeps stirring up a lot of feelings inside us, it is one of life's taps on the shoulder – an inner call, if you like, to look inside and listen to what these feelings are trying to tell us. I have often heard women who have been diagnosed with cancer speak about their 'wounds of love'. This occurs particularly in those with breast cancer but is also said by women who have other of the female cancers. I have also heard many women say,

'It seems a ridiculous thing to say, but I'm grateful in lots of ways for my cancer. It has forced me to look at my life and the things that have happened to me. As a result of this my life has more depth, meaning and passion. If I hadn't had cancer I don't think I would have ever seen life this way.'

For most of us, though, our invitation to look inside comes via our feelings of hurt, pain, anger or indifference that are our soul's call for help. I believe that women need to hear a new story about sex in middle and old age. Most of what I have read gives me good information, helps ease the fear, and puts into context a great deal of the physical and some of the emotional backdrop to this stage of life. There are deep and profound feelings around ageing, loss and mortality that certainly need the integrity of time and space as well as the safety of being listened to and validated. But there is still a gap. The soul thirsts.

With time *love* becomes the vehicle for launching vast creative powers of transformation and deep wisdom.

When I was in my thirties I read and heard a lot being said about 'the wisdom that comes with the middle years'. Now, twenty years later, as I listen to women in their midlife, what I hear are stories of hurt and disappointed dreams. The Promised Land of wise women seems tantalisingly just out of reach. The painful feelings of hurt and disappointment are often turned inwards into bitterness and cynicism. Issues around sex become the arena where this crescendo of emotion and feeling frequently finds its catharsis. A woman's heart aches; her sensuality is numbed like that of a child who has sobbed herself to sleep. But there is a healing power that lies hidden deep within this wound. Correctly perceived and respectfully experienced, this wound can be truly sacred and can generate a new fertility. As Jean Houston writes in *The Search for the Beloved*, 'With time *love* becomes the vehicle for launching vast creative powers of transformation and deep wisdom.'

As I sit and listen to a woman share her pain, there seems to be a recurring story at the root of her sobbing. She has led a parallel existence with her husband. Both roughly head in the same direction, but rarely touch. She hasn't been listened to; she feels unimportant and taken for granted. She has brought up the family, and has been the entertainer, mother confessor, chief cook and bottle washer – all things to all people. But somehow, in the middle of all this activity, deep inside she feels untouched, unseen and lonely. Something different is needed to awaken the senses, like early morning dew on the night's sleeping grass. The heart needs tender cradling in love's caring bosom. The soul aches to be pulled deeper into a period of healing and renewal, much the same way as the caterpillar is drawn into a metamorphosis inside a chrysalis. Within the chrysalis the power of human love can melt us, mould us, heal us, and transform us.

It often takes a while for the light to go on and for us to realise that all the searching and wrestling we do with people on the outside arises from our pain and fear and a feeling of being separate and alone. Therefore, all solutions begin with the return journey to reconnect to the boundless love which resides deep within.

I remember Sarah, who met her husband, Tim, while they were at university. They were both madly in love and wanted to get married. Their parents were adamant that this was ridiculous as Tim still had three years to go of a medical degree, and at least a year of horrendous hours of residency and, during all this, no money. Sarah had two years of her accounting degree to finish when they decided to marry. She left her studies and took a job as a bookkeeper to support them both while Tim finished his degree.

When I met up with them 30 years later she was bitter and resentful, felt bad about herself and said, 'Sex, that's the very last thing on my list of life's priorities! I'm battling to survive in here, on my own as usual.' Tim was now a prominent, successful, wealthy and well-respected surgeon. He had a generous social conscience and gave time, money and expertise to causes in need. He was personable, likeable, and had done his best, he said, 'to look after Sarah and the kids and give them what we had to struggle so hard for when we were young.'

However Sarah and Tim were in trouble. They were not communicating. When they came for counselling their first challenge was to learn how to create a place of emotional safety with each other so they could begin to speak honestly. They were first asked to tell each other two things they appreciated about each other. One of the surest ways to start building safety is for partners to agree to cut out all criticism, attack and blame.

For example, instead of Sarah saying, 'Tim you are so messy', I encouraged her to say, 'I feel resentful when the kitchen is left in a mess.' For them to be really honest and vulnerable with each other it was absolutely vital for them to maintain safety (see Chapter 2). Tim and Sarah had not felt safe together. They described it as 'like treading on eggshells around each other'. She felt taken for granted and not listened to. He felt criticised. Neither felt it was possible to be intimate emotionally. She certainly didn't feel like making love and he resented that. But even animals in the wild will not mate if they feel unsafe.

In the process of the dialogues Sarah and Tim had with each other, Sarah discovered that she had unconsciously internalised a huge part of her mother's story. The end result was her feeling very resentful towards anyone with competence and power.

'I can't believe I have spent all my life deliberately trying to be the exact opposite of my mother. And I am exactly like her! Now I can see I'm living out her feelings!'

It was a powerful realisation for Sarah. 'I feel a huge relief already! If I can do something inside myself to feel better and I don't have to try and change Tim, that's simple!'

If a woman is feeling trapped in feelings of inadequacy, resentment and pain there is no point talking to her about love and wisdom. I am reminded of a saying by the Chinese philosopher, Chuang Tzu: 'A frog in a well cannot be talked to about the sea.'

For this precise reason I often say to women, 'Begin with a little bit of patience with yourself and just take baby steps.' All you need is a little willingness to start, and a lot of wanting to be happy and have inner peace.

There are four stages of this metamorphosis from caterpillar to butterfly:

1. **Forgiveness** This means letting go of old stories carried in your head of unresolved hurts, angers and resentment from the past.
2. **The gymnasium** Physical, emotional and spiritual muscles need strengthening to prepare for the journey.
3. **Awakening** This requires listening and making friends with the woman inside.
4. **Wisdom** This occurs by forming a relationship with self, with others, and with soul.

Forgiveness

Forgiveness is the key to feelings of self-worth, happiness and inner peace. It is an important practice all through life, but at midlife forgiveness is essential, because failing to do this will leave us very vulnerable to depression.

Forgiveness is letting go of old stories that have their roots in a history of sadness, betrayal, abandonment and grief. Make no mistake, these stories were lived out by real live characters. Imagine a woman with four hungry mouths to feed. It is during the Great Depression and her husband has no job. With his self-esteem shot to pieces, he drinks away the little money they have. No wonder she thinks 'men are no-hopers' and passes that message on to her children. The stories are handed down from one generation to the next and 'eat us up' with anger and bitterness. But we can no longer afford to pay the enormous cost to our health and happiness (see Chapter 26 on forgiveness).

Although they appear funny at first hearing, some of the one-line quips and urban myths about 'what men are' and 'what women are' have a sting in their tail that numbs the longing for closeness that deep down we all share.

Women need a guiding story to hold them in the 'rite of passage' of midlife. We need credible role models who inspire us to find another way – a way that nourishes us and gives us hope and courage to choose new responses to old situations.

Here is an exercise to try.

Becoming aware of the belief systems of your parents

- Sit in a comfortable chair and imagine that you are your mother.
- Sit like her, breathe like her, and feel into her emotions.
- Now imagine that she is speaking through you and have her complete the following statements:

  'Women are ....'

  'Men are ....'

  'Sex is ....'

  Now do the same exercise with your father.

We often carry around the stories and belief systems of our parents without even being aware of it. Our parents' life stories become like self-fulfilling prophecies that find expression in our life. They often shape and control our lives without our awareness.

You may wonder what this has to do with your own sexuality. Ask yourself the questions:

'Do I want to be right or do I want to be happy?'

'Are the stories in my head helping me or hindering me?'

'What is the self-talk I hear in my head about sex, my body, his body, what I want, what he wants?'

We really need to let go of past ways. Our generation has seen the introduction of the contraceptive 'pill', the sexual revolution, the feminist revolution, the nuclear family, the single-parent family, and women are now taking their equal place in the workforce. We cannot look in the rear-vision mirror using old stories to sustain us as we move forward into the future. The modern woman needs a new story because the old ones don't seem to hold her or give her hope. They tend to sour her, harden her and cause her pain. She hardened originally as a reaction to protect herself from getting hurt again. Now her hardness has become a sarcophagus, keeping her in the illusion of safety. But instead of safety, it actually encases her in her own agony where the worms of bitterness eat at her dreams.

By letting go of the old stories, we make it possible for the healing power of love and grace to enter the chrysalis.

Sarah and Tim certainly needed a new way of looking at what was happening to them if their marriage of 30 years was going to survive. Sarah was the oldest in her family, with a younger brother and sister. Her father owned a small business and worked, literally, from dawn till dusk and later. Money was always tight, but all the children were given the opportunity of an education and she has memories of a few family holidays.

Her mother stayed at home, made all their clothes, and took in some sewing for friends. She did a lot of sewing for the church and the children's schools. She was a very hard-working, loving woman but felt very inadequate, taking things home to sew rather than doing canteen and other things because she did not feel as good as the other women at the schools. She left school when she was fourteen to help out with a large family.

When I asked Sarah what her mother thought of sex she laughed wryly and said, 'As little as possible. It was another of the duties she needed to perform. I think she found it quite distasteful, but they were happy enough, so I guess she didn't mind if it kept him happy.' Although Sarah had had a good education she felt it was inferior to Tim's. She felt inadequate alongside him and carried the same feelings of inferiority as her mother. She never felt totally comfortable taking her rightful place at his side. Because she didn't feel good about herself, she tried very hard to please and then became very resentful when she perceived this as being unnoticed and unappreciated. They had never really learned to communicate honestly so it followed inevitably that with waning hormones sex became a real problem, just as it had for her mother.

When Sarah understood how much of her mother's story she had internalised and lived out, she felt huge relief. She had always known that she was a lot like her mother; in fact, she had spent a lot of energy deliberately doing the exact opposite of anything her mother did. To fully experience how much her mother's story was still at work in her life brought both shock and relief. She was certainly very ready to let this 'old' story go. She wanted to forgive her mother and herself. In addition, with the new level of honesty in their communication, Sarah and Tim were beginning to feel close again, 'just like when we first met'.

The gymnasium

This is the chrysalis stage, a time of preparation and strengthening for this very important stage of life transformation. Here, a routine of some form of exercise and meditation and/or prayer is essential to:

- develop an attitude of gratitude
- be thankful for all the people and situations in your life, both joyful and painful
- practise releasing attachment to problems – worrying does not make them better
- stop all criticism – it only makes you feel miserable.

This is central because a woman has to prepare herself for 'the change', not just in her body but also in her heart and her soul. Everything she will be called upon to do inside herself during this transformation will require strength and focus and will at times feel like it is all too much. But in my experience women have magnificent powers of strength they can call upon.

I watch our oldest daughter, Lahra, as she channels enormous strength and focus on a daily basis. Like most young mothers with two babies, she has to get up night after night and gets very little sleep. Sometimes this goes on for weeks on end with feeding, teething or colds happening with one or the other. Being sleep deprived becomes a way of life. After a full and busy day with a preschooler and a one-year-old, just to get through the 'four o'clock frenzies' and get them bathed, fed and into bed is an incredible feat. Lahra, like other mothers, repeats this day after day with a warm delight in her babies and a magnificent creative strength. If I were to ask her to reflect on what she was doing, she would laugh at me quizzically. But make no mistake: she is building reserves, like a squirrel gathering nuts for winter. She is building a vast reservoir of strength that can be called upon for the rest of her life. Her brain, and even her muscles, will carry the memory of how to focus and push through when nothing inside wants to or feels like it. But she needs to do it for a greater good.

Perhaps Lahra's story will remind you of a magnificent part of yourself that you had forgotten. Take a look back over your life and make a list of the times when that one inside (you) has appeared like an inner strength and pulled you through despite difficulty or adversity – times when, on looking back, you don't know how you did it. As with Lahra, very ordinary, but at the same time extraordinary.

Great numbers of women pass through the midlife rite of passage. In many ways it is reminiscent of childbirth. It can be painful but has enormous rewards. We can avoid a lot of the complications by having a willingness to 'go with the flow'. Just as in childbirth, when we experienced the painful contractions around *change* in our lives, it does not mean something has gone wrong. Pain is often an integral part of change.

For us to successfully negotiate this midlife passage, the more willing we are to change the better. We will be called on to be willing to *change* our relationship with ourselves, with our world and with the people who are close to us in our world. Finally, we will be called on to *change* our relationship with the power of love and grace in our hearts and our lives.

As indicated, other stages in life are marked by ritual and preparation. But midlife seeps into our awareness and one day we wake up and say, 'I don't feel like I used to – what's happened?' If you look back at your life, you will see that in each of the preceding stages in which you made changes, you were helped by people, by stories, by celebration and by rituals. As I watched the Sydney Olympics on television in 2000 there was a real sense of Australia coming of age. This was due, in part, to the proud telling of our nation's stories during the opening and closing ceremonies. We 'baby boomers' really need stories to help us feel proud of who we are and what we have achieved. We also need to feel a sense of quiet satisfaction and graceful integrity with our own 'coming of age'. Just reflect on all the years of *preparation* that went into making the Sydney Olympics such an amazing event.

The awakening

The third stage involves learning how to make our body a 'good friend' we can relax with. This entails work within the chrysalis and tapping into the archetypal powers of awakening the woman who has missed a vital stage in her development. I have seen some women who have left home to get married and moved from being a child to a wife without ever having been a woman. It's as if they know how to be a child and then how to become a mother, but have *never been a woman*.

Healing our attitude to our body is central to our happiness ... It has been thin and fat, looked at, measured and compared. It needs our unconditional love.

Sometimes in our history, as a result of life's tragedies, it was a mother or a grandmother whose inner woman went to sleep several generations back. The story might be something like that of a grandmother who, as a young girl, was forbidden by her family to marry the boy she loved, and then was forced into a marriage with a man *she* didn't love, but of whom the family approved. The woman inside her closed down in grief and remains still deep inside women in her line two generations later.

Or there may be stored hurts around the vulnerable time of pregnancy and childbirth. The early weeks and months after giving birth is such a tender period. Women are very open and vulnerable at this time and an act of thoughtlessness by their partner will go very deep. Women so often bring up the pain around these incidents 30 years later. The pain needs to be talked about and cleared because it often gets in the way of her being happy and sexually alive.

Catherine was 50 when she and her husband, Bill, came to see me. They described 'one of their horror patches', which had intermittently plagued them all through their 23 years of marriage. These were usually precipitated by Bill hurting Catherine in some way, either intentionally or unintentionally, by 'trying to control me'. Catherine would then withdraw and 'be a good girl and try and please in order to keep the peace'. This in turn caused her to feel very resentful towards Bill.

Bill mentioned that he was getting fed up with Catherine's rituals around home safety, which had been triggered by an incident six months previously. A friend of Catherine's from her bridge club had been savagely attacked by a prowler who had broken into her home in the early hours of the morning. In her fear Catherine turned her home into 'Fort Knox' with everything locked and alarmed, both day and night. Bill finally spat the dummy when she wanted to fit a large bolt to the inside of the bedroom door to keep them 'safe' while they slept.

Catherine added to this story by saying that for all their marriage she had never been comfortable getting undressed with the light on or the door open. Since the friend's house break-in, the discomfort had increased to such an extent that she had to lock herself in the bathroom to get changed. Sex always needed to be at night with the lights out and

Catherine was much more comfortable wearing a nightie or some form of clothing to cover her body even while making love.

When I asked Catherine what feelings she had when she thought of her naked body, she thought for a while and said 'mainly fear, shame and guilt, and I suppose a little bit of anger'. She had been sexually abused by her stepfather from age seven to fourteen. He had a military background and regimented the whole family by being angry and controlling and going into fits of rage when he had been drinking. He would come into her room late at night and ask her to get out of bed while he watched her as she took off her pyjamas.

After some time in therapy, Catherine started to feel her anger, revulsion and contempt towards her stepfather and began to see the connection between this man and what was happening in her relationship with Bill, as well as the connection to her need for safety.

In time she was able to free her relationship with Bill and her present life from the experiences of her childhood, and began to feel a genuine compassion towards her stepfather. However, her huge obstacle was facing the denial or 'blindness' of her mother. How come she didn't know? If she did, why didn't she do something to protect her? How could a woman let that happen to another woman, let alone her very own daughter? For Catherine, this was the ultimate betrayal and the deepest wound, which had affected her attitude towards herself as a woman, and underpinned the shame and guilt with which she viewed her body.

Months later, when she reflected on how lovingly she had cared for, protected and championed her three daughters she felt an overwhelming sense of being redeemed and her self-respect being returned. She said, 'I've had a hand guiding me. Alone, I would never have been able to do such a fantastic job of raising my children.' She paused, and then with a huge smile of satisfaction, said: 'I am a fantastic mother.' I added, 'and you are a wonderful and courageous woman'.

Healing our attitude to our body is central to our happiness. There is nothing that we have evaluated, criticised and judged more than our own body. This body has been our most intimate home. If we are mothers, it has carried, given life to and nurtured our babies. It has endured sickness, health, surgery and recovery. It has been thin and fat, looked at, measured and compared. It needs our unconditional love. We really need to ask forgiveness for all the judgements and criticism and begin to appreciate it just as it is. You may wish to write a letter to your body and ask for forgiveness, and then look in the mirror and say 'Thank you'.

It takes time for metamorphosis inside the chrysalis before awakening is possible. It is during this stage of metamorphosis that you must ask yourself the questions:

'How much do I really want to be happy, fully alive, in love, sensual, spiritual, a power for good (and I would add, a power for God)?'
'Am I willing to take the extraordinary action necessary to achieve this?'
'If I neglect to do this, what is the price I will have to pay?'

Part of this third stage is commitment – commitment to yourself, to union with a deeper part of you. I call it 'soul'. If you are not intimate with yourself, how can you be intimate with anyone else? Because women have spent such a huge amount of their lives being aware of everyone else, to start listening to themselves can feel quite strange and awkward. I often hear women speak of a feeling of naivety, innocence and newness when moving through simple things such as 'What music do I like?' 'What sort of food do I like to cook?' 'What time do I like to go to bed?' to the more profound, such as simply listening to the longing in their hearts. They are unused to feeling so in touch with themselves.

The untapped potential of a mature woman is formidable. She has strength and focus; she has practicality and endurance. Particularly if she has been a mother, she is quite practised at getting the 'I' out of the centre of her thoughts. This will put her in a state of readiness for other parts of her life to be entered into and experienced in their fullness. All these realisations can unfold within the still space of the chrysalis. *This is the awakening.*

Wisdom

Early steps outside the chrysalis have to do with balance. One of the constants in my life is trying to keep in balance a number of things that are important to me: relationship, prayer/meditation, work, fun, exercise, being of service, to name a few. I am constantly trying to balance the inner and the outer.

Look for your gifts or blessings. A wonderful nun who taught me at school used to say, 'We are all gifts and are blessed with miracles to pass on; we just need to exercise them.' Here are some you may relate to:

- Some of us are filled with an appreciation of nature; share it.
- Some are blessed with laughter; laugh lots with people around you.
- Some of us have a keen sense of justice; speak about it.
- Others are blessed with compassion; express it.
- Some of us have a capacity for awe and wonder at the stars at night or the beauty in people: share, share, share it.

We don't have a full appreciation of our 'gifts' until we share them with others. Being of service creates warmth and joy and expands your world with miracles.

Give permission for your heart and soul to be healed. Decide you will no longer find value in resentment, anger and criticism. Blame reinforces powerlessness (see 'Take charge of your choices' in Chapter 2). In other words, 'Be a love finder not a fault finder.' This is one of the principles of Attitudinal Healing (see Chapter 27).

Our minds are like computers. What we program in is what we will get out. Most of us wouldn't put toxic abusive substances in our body, but we don't give a second thought to putting all sorts of critical abusive thoughts into our head. Women (and men too) are defined by the quality of their relationships.

You now have the tools for an intimate relationship with yourself – the beloved inside you. That is why I have left it until now to speak directly about sex.

For a woman, sex without the context of relationship is meaningless. As mentioned previously, there is no point in trying to have a relationship with someone else if you don't have an intimate connection with yourself.

We need to clear our minds of old stories and scripts that serve no useful purpose. This includes, of course, letting go of the resentments that have lived rent-free in our heads for so long. What a relief when we do! It's really worth the effort of becoming good at this sort of mental spring-cleaning. It makes us so much more available for 'lovemaking' in all its different forms. I believe that lovemaking is first and foremost soul-making. When we are at home with ourselves, physical lovemaking with another takes on a fuller, richer quality. It is not 'giving in', or doing what someone else wants us to do, but rather an invitation to communion with our own being. From that fertile base can spring a wonderful assortment of passion, excitement, discovery and pleasure. And, of course, we all know what effect that can have on a tired relationship.

As women we need relationships, both inner and outer, as a context within which to discover and express our identity and meaning. Physical love-making is one important expression of our ever-developing sexuality. It can be a rich, enjoyable and deeply fulfilling expression of our love.

Life, in the form of relationships, continuously offers us an invitation to connect with our soul and to the beloved within.

Summary

- For a woman, sexuality is intrinsically connected to her relationship with her partner, her self-worth and her soul.
- Before a woman can express herself and her sexuality creatively, she must have an intimate relationship with herself.
- For women in midlife struggling with hurt, anger and resentment, there are ways to heal themselves.
- What is required is letting go of negative stories from the past; physical, emotional and spiritual strengthening; making friends with the woman inside; and finally, forming a relationship with self, with other and with soul.
- Once we have reached this stage, physical lovemaking will become an expression of our love in all its beauty.

21

Lost zest; reward offered –
how testosterone can help

There is nothing so powerful as a menopausal woman with zest.

Margaret Mead (1901–1978), Anthropologist

Zest can be expressed in many ways. Zest is about having positive feelings. But to lose one's overall zest for living is a tragedy. As one woman put it sadly, 'My get up and go has got up and gone!' For her, it was her sexual energy as much as her general physical energy.

We see women crippled by arthritis, or bent double by osteoporosis. These physical afflictions certainly decrease physical and mental energy and are hard to bear. They are related to menopause and may be helped by HRT. Saddest of all, however, is when emotional energy drains away. The best definition of depression that I know is 'absence of joy' and it includes absence of zest also. Using HRT may help, but life events and attitudes are the major factors in determining emotional energy around midlife.

There is now adequate help for physical and emotional symptoms of menopause, but when sexual energy declines, or disappears, a woman may be reluctant to discuss this, especially with a male doctor. Even if she does bring up the subject she may be told that nothing can be done

– 'You will just have to live with it' (actually meaning *without* it!). So in this chapter we focus mainly on the loss of sexual energy caused by menopause.

Once again it is important to emphasise that not all loss of sexual interest is hormonal. And we need to distinguish between libido (desire for or wanting sex) and performance and sexual response.

It does not seem to be generally known that women produce significant amounts of male hormones from their ovaries, as well as from the adrenal glands, throughout life. Even when ovaries fail to produce female hormones, because all the eggs have gone, other cells in the ovaries produce testosterone. This explains why old ladies lose their feminine curves and may grow facial hair. (We have often heard it said that as some men age they turn into old women, so the reverse also seems to be true.) Men produce significant amounts of estrogens as well as large amounts of testosterone throughout life. Men who are alcoholics, and whose livers are failing, will often have significant breast enlargement because the liver can no longer metabolise these estrogens. The *balance* of hormones is what is important for both men and women.

In recent years medical researchers, particularly Professor Susan Davis, have investigated the role of the male hormone, testosterone, in pre- and postmenopausal women. In a study reported in 1999, Davis showed that administering testosterone via a patch to premenopausal women with low testosterone levels relieved many of the symptoms that had been named premenstrual syndrome (PMS), i.e. lowered mood and irritability, as well as loss of libido and general energy.

Similarly, I have noted that although estrogen replacement may relieve the classic deficiency symptoms, it may not always restore general energy and zest, or full sexual functioning (including libido), in women at menopause. In my practice I usually measure the testosterone level if symptoms suggest it may be low. It has long been my practice to replace testosterone (using subcutaneous implants) in *young* women who have been castrated, i.e. had both ovaries removed because of disease such as endometriosis, severe pelvic inflammatory disease or pelvic cancer. But testosterone deficiency in normal postmenopausal women has been largely ignored, mainly because there have been no testosterone products available to use. Injections containing estrogen and testosterone were available for a few years, but were taken off the market, probably because there was so little demand for them. Currently, in Australia, testosterone cream is available only in Western Australia, and patches are not available in any states. Women and their doctors are understandably wary about using male hormones in women because of the known side effects of masculinisation, such as deepening of the voice, hair growth (especially facial), and increased muscle bulk (helpful for athletes but not for feminine women). These effects are related, usually, to a high or prolonged dosage of testosterone.

Judy is aged 52. She had a relatively easy menopause with few flushes or other problems. She has recently remarried and loves her new husband deeply. Her first marriage terminated in a messy divorce five years ago. Sex was unsatisfactory for the last ten years of that marriage. Her husband was unfaithful and blamed her lack of sexual response for his defection, but she confided that he was a very unsatisfactory lover so that her needs were hardly ever met. She therefore had simply switched off and no longer loved him. She had no sexual partner for the next three years. Now her vagina is dry, but this she has been able to overcome with lubricants. Her sexual response is very slow or absent. Her new husband is extremely patient, but this only makes her feel worse because her very real love for him does not result in any satisfying sexual response. Hormone measurement revealed a very low level of testosterone as well as low estrogen.

Vaginal estrogens were prescribed to help the vaginal dryness and she was given testosterone cream, as well as a combined hormone patch (estrogen and progesterone) in a low dose to be used on a continuous basis. Within two months she reported a return of libido, comfortable intercourse and an improvement in general energy.

It is not good practice to give testosterone alone without estrogen to balance it, so although she had no significant estrogen deficiency symptoms Judy was given low-dose estrogen as well as progestogen – the latter to protect the uterus against abnormal bleeding (see Chapter 11, 'To bleed or not to bleed, that is the question'). I can understand that women may feel doubtful about the need to protect the uterus as if estrogens are dangerous, possibly cancer-inducing, 'drugs'. Estrogens are not drugs, although they are produced in a laboratory. The main estrogen in use these days, particularly in patches, is pure, *natural* estradiol. This is identical to the hormone that the ovary produces in such quantity during reproductive life. Estrone, the main constituent of Premarin (which is extracted from the urine of pregnant mares and is the most widely used estrogen in the USA), is also, in a sense, a natural hormone, being the same as the hormone produced by our adrenal glands when the ovaries fail. But Premarin contains other estrogenic substances such as equilinin, which may be natural to the horse but not necessarily to women.

> **It is not good practice to give testosterone alone without estrogen to balance it ...**

Much of the estrone is converted, in the body, into estradiol. However, measuring estrogen levels in the blood when a woman is on oral HRT may give a false idea of how much estrogen is actually available to the body, since we do not measure estrone but only estradiol. (This is for technical reasons as the estrone assay is difficult and expensive to do, and so is only done for research purposes.) The blood level of estradiol in a woman using a patch or estrogen implants, or certain oral therapies, *is* an accurate measurement of the estrogen available because the hormone that is being given is being measured.

Not all postmenopausal women suffer from deficiency of testosterone as well as estrogen, so I do not believe that testosterone needs replacing unless there are specific symptoms such as low libido, low energy levels, and unexplained lowering of mood and blood levels of testosterone confirming a deficiency. These symptoms may appear before menopause and be blamed on other things such as PMS (see Chapter 8, 'War and peace – menstrual mayhem and PMS') or depression (see Chapter 16). Again, it may be both. If it is hormonal, it may be possible to truly restore sexual and physical zest. Remember, 'there is nothing so powerful as a menopausal woman with zest'.

A recent study published in the July 2005 issue of the *Journal of the American Medical Association* says that there is no correlation between androgen (male hormone) levels and sexual function in women. In the article Professor Susan Davis reported the results of a recent study in Victoria and concluded that 'Evidence that a low serum testosterone level distinguishes women with low sexual function from others and that androgen deficiency syndrome can be identified biochemically is lacking'. However, she qualified this by saying that the results of her own study were not in conflict with testosterone being used pharmacologically for hypo-active sexual desire.

It would appear from all this that the jury is still out!

Summary

- Losing one's zest for life is tragic.
- Lack of zest is often expressed in a decline in sexual as well as physical energy, which is sometimes caused by lack of testosterone in women in midlife.
- Administering a testosterone patch or cream may help in alleviating the symptoms of low mood, lack of energy and libido if the problem is hormonal. It is even possible that this will restore both physical and sexual zest, although research opinions are mixed.

22

Men and menopause

A woman marries a man expecting he will change but he doesn't. A man marries a woman expecting that she won't change and she does!

Anon

Although *menopause* is *women's* business and there is no direct male equivalent, this does not let men off the hook. They can participate more willingly in the female menopause and along the way learn to be grateful that they are spared much of the direct hormonal turmoil.

As noted above, a man expects that a woman will *not* change, but she does, and often he can't deal with the change. The greatest change of all for the woman, the menopause, often alienates him. Men's hormones do fade away as they age, but it is a gradual process, usually without a cliff edge over which to fall, so it is not surprising that they do not understand a lot of what is happening to women. They do not have a hormonal menopause as women do, but many do go through a midlife crisis, which may occur at the same time. In reality, many women go through male menopause as well as female menopause because they often lose their male hormones as well as their female ones.

The main aim of this chapter is to give men a chance to understand what some women go through, so that they can provide support rather than criticism. Menopause can be a time of reckoning for them, too, and an opportunity for change.

Men's reactions to the changes at menopause are varied and not always helpful:

- A few men do try to understand and give support.
- Some switch off, pretending nothing is happening (don't rock the boat).
- Some turn their backs and walk out.
- Some trade their old-model partner for a newer shiny one.

Menopause can be a time of reckoning for [men], and an opportunity for change. Men are under increasing pressure these days. They are expected to be there in the labour ward, and to participate in a way that would have shocked their fathers who would have said, 'Having babies is women's business.' Now the baby boomers are expecting their men to be around for menopause also – not to participate directly of course, but to be sympathetic and aware. For many men the change in their partners is baffling.

Some men bring 'the wife' to me to be fixed up, as if she were a car that had broken down or needed a new battery. They would like her to have a Viagra-type 'fix' for her disappearing sex drive. As I take a careful history, I sometimes find that it is the relationship that needs fixing rather than just her sex drive.

One of my patients sent me a note: 'Have you ever noticed that all of our problems begin with MEN? Mental anxiety, mental breakdown, menstrual cramps, menopause.'

Another patient, Felicity, sent me this frank account of her midlife relationship crisis.

I am writing this to you, as one of your menopausal patients, in the hope that it may give heart to someone else.

I am an intelligent, well-educated, well-read, well-travelled woman who was in the workforce for many years and I still accepted such nonsense about myself as a woman! During the months that I have been out there in the wilderness trying to sort myself out, I have been overwhelmed by the understanding and support that I have received from those I have confided in. My similar age girlfriends, my 86-year-old aunt, and even my daughters were never judgemental, just there to listen and wait for me to find my answer. Note that all these were women. Attempts to explain how I was feeling to my husband fell on deaf ears.

I had an amazing love affair: an instant attraction to a man I met at one dinner and then a subsequent lunch. He pursued me across the world and it gave me such a buzz. My sexuality returned with such a bang that it is now making my marriage worthwhile. It also made me consider how much we blame on menopause. I'm not at all sad that it happened. It was so wonderful to have a charming man pursue me across the world. I'm sure that my disinterest in sex in my marriage was a result of boredom, which seems to happen only too often in long-term relationships, and not just as a result of the onset of menopause. Meeting this man jolted me out of my doldrums and, gradually, as I worked out what I wanted with my life, it has given me the impetus to improve what hasn't been successful in my marriage during many years. So that's what I am working on.

Because my husband has always been loving and caring, it made me sad that he could not really understand what I was trying to tell him about my feelings at midlife. We are completing a lovely house in the country to which we will be moving permanently. My life, despite all my illnesses, has been satisfying. I am able to pursue my artwork at my own pace, having my own studio to work in. I have a wonderful relationship with both of my grown-up daughters, my son-in-law and two grandsons. To jeopardise all this for someone I met at a lunch and one dinner seemed totally crazy!

I finally came to the conclusion that I could not play deceitful games for a prolonged period, however flattering it was to be pursued. So, after much soul searching, I opted out (maybe that should read 'chickened out'). Yes, my husband did know something, but just how much I am not sure. One day I hope I will be able to talk to him about it. He is, after all, my best friend.

———

Tina told me: 'I find myself being disappointed in men. In 32 years of marriage I've learnt to shut up when he is upset. When he had cooled down then it was my turn, but he usually did not stay to listen to what I had to say anyway. I have decided that, at this time of life, it is my turn to speak first, but he *still* does not stay around to listen. I wasn't heard then, and I'm not heard now. *No wonder I am frustrated.* I want to kick him where it hurts most.'

Liz said, 'Bill is so charming: everyone says that he's such a *caring* man. So when I begin to feel grotty and unstable he pats me on the head, with a smile, and says, "There there, go and buy yourself a new dress, I'm sure it will all pass." I'm too hot and sweaty to buy a new dress. I want to take all my clothes off and lie under a fan. I certainly don't want to be patted down. *And it isn't funny!*'

Gail said, 'All my expectations have ended in disappointment. *I've really had to earn my happiness.* I have been waiting for the time when there would be just us. With the kids gone I thought we could go out more, have friends in, or have a really good holiday. But Eric just wants to watch TV. He's sports mad. I can't compete with the football and the golf and the soccer – and now it's the cricket.

'I turned the TV off the other night so that I could talk to him. I tried to tell him how I was feeling at the moment, that I just want to be loved. I'm having some flushes and my moods are up and down, but I mostly just feel sad. I'm sad that we two do not have much as a couple any more. He looked at me as if I had gone crazy and said, "Go and see your doctor and get yourself back together", then turned the TV back on. *When is he ever going to hear what I am saying?*'

Sandra says: 'We've been married for 26 years. Graeme has a very short fuse. I usually just give in, but lately I've begun to think, "Why should I?" He has been avoiding sex for nearly a year. When I tried to talk to him about it he refused to discuss it. I met a man at our local tennis club who was the exact opposite of Graeme. I found I could talk to him. We had an affair. Of course Graeme found out. The affair was over, anyway, and I had not intended to leave the marriage. *I was desperate for someone to talk to*. I asked for forgiveness, but now Graeme uses the affair against me whenever we have the slightest disagreement. I feel blackmailed.

'We went to a workshop on menopause and premenopause. He asked a lot of questions and then made an appointment for me to see one of the doctors. I didn't really want to go because I think *he* needs help even more than *I* do. When we went to that doctor he tried to do all the talking. He just took over, as usual. Then the doctor asked him to let me answer the questions. By this stage I felt so angry that I just wanted to leave, but somehow the doctor cottoned on to the real problem and began to talk to Graeme more about *his* sexual problem. I've started on a low dose of HRT for my hot flushes and Graeme has agreed to see a specialist. Whether he goes or not, I feel to even get this far is something new in our relationship. We are talking to each other a lot more about everything and he has stopped blackmailing me.

'I really think that men have a sort of menopause, but they can't or don't know how to talk about it.'

Ivy says: 'Men and their mothers! That dragon mother-in-law of mine who, of course, just breezed through menopause, thinks I'm a wimp! She also had seven children and dropped them like you'd expect a bitch to. I had trouble with both of mine, so of course I'm not much of a mother either in her eyes. My father-in-law is switched off. It's the only way he has been able to survive! I'm having hot flushes and I cry at the drop of a hat. My husband says I'm overreacting. He has no patience with me at all. *Sometimes I'd like to go and sit in the dog kennel and get away from all the critics.* My mother died of breast cancer at menopause so I don't know what else she went through and I'm rather scared to try HRT.'

Julienne says: 'My vagina is dry. Intercourse often leaves me screaming with pain. He never asks me why. I'm sure my husband thinks it's because *he* is so good sexually!'

I'm always glad when men come with their wives to seminars on midlife. Even a little learning, rather than being dangerous, is helpful in this instance. I think that learning needs to be fun, not a catalogue of medical facts. Patricia and I, with her husband Donatus, have run several 'brain sex' seminars where we demonstrate the very real differences between male and female experiences and responses. It is also helpful if you can talk freely with other women who are going through similar struggles and feeling alone and helpless. This book, also, will give you a chance to read other women's experiences and realise that you are not suffering alone and that there is help available. In Chapter 20, 'Sexuality and your relationship – in need of the beloved', we discussed these issues and gave some simple steps to change and enrich your relationship.

Men may also experience change of life and a midlife crisis, but it is not a true menopause as occurs in women, who have definite cessation of hormone production and loss of fertility. Some men would like to think that menopause is to blame for all sexual and relationship difficulties around midlife. Hormonal deficiency will certainly cause local pain due to vaginal dryness and decline in sexual responses with the loss of both oestrogens and testosterone, but men must take some responsibility for relationship difficulties. For *most* of the women I quote in this chapter there is a hormonal problem and it may well be lack of both male and female hormones, but the problem is compounded by their partners' disinterest. Men need help to understand their partners' crises and perhaps their own.

Affairs and abandonment

For some women, one of the great wounds occurs when their husband or partner has affairs and/or leaves them for another woman. The sense of shame, humiliation and inadequacy they feel seems to strike at the very heart of what it means to be a woman. It is a love wound that plummets them into the depths of shame and abandonment. They talk about, 'The ripping agony that tears at your guts when you experience your man's eyes passing you by as if you didn't exist' and 'The experience of your womb dropping through your body's floor as you watch him focus on another.'

Like all the great wounds of the psyche this wound is an invitation into soul-making.

Soul-making happens when the wounding is so profound it splits us open, and new questions begin to be asked about who we are at our core. The paradox is that by entering fully into the turmoil a new energy, a quiet but powerful surety, emerges. In the fullness of truth our wounding is an invitation into our renaissance. This process has a life of its own. However much we would like to skip over or hurry through the different stages, because they tumble us into the pits of our pain and neurosis, the process cannot be hurried. Each stage takes its own time and must be treated with its own integrity.

The stages of fear, anger, shame, humiliation, abandonment, betrayal, rage, vengeance, loneliness and grief are all part of the story that must be felt and entered into. There is a chaos of feelings and stages. They can be experienced one at a time or all at the same time, and there is no order of difficulty. When you can put it into the context of a larger story, you can begin to see into the midst of the chaos.

The suffering cracks the boundaries of what you thought you could bear. The force of this wounding pierces the shell of the being you thought you were. In the breaking open of the old way, we begin to move in new directions and see things that had been hidden to us previously. In much the same way as when the sperm pierces the ovum, it is the beginning of another, larger reality. Most religious traditions and many of our great stories from mythology give us a context for viewing this birth, this death and finally this rebirth.

At times of pain and crises like these, we feel bewildered and confused. We ask ourselves, 'Is what I thought was real merely an illusion after all?' When our defences are down we are more vulnerable and thus more open and available to be reached by larger forces of grace and healing. Correctly perceived, this can be a time of great transformation and personal growth. As a car bumper sticker I once read proclaimed, 'I worked very hard to have this nervous breakdown, so now I'm going to enjoy it!' Our psyche has pulled this towards us as an opportunity for transformation. Instead of fighting against the change, we can learn to embrace it. The pain is not less but the consequence more profound and whole. The wounding breaks open the recognised boundaries within which we have made our world.

The strange beauty that can emerge from this 'sacred' wounding is that we get in touch with a new reality. What is happening? This wounding is not something that has gone wrong. It can lead us to ask the questions, 'Why is this happening to me?' and 'What can I learn from all this?'

I remember attending a series of lectures by Fr Richard Rohr, a Franciscan priest from the United States. He invited us to embrace our painful experiences, to enter into the belly of the whale, like Jonah in the Old Testament. As he spoke I experienced a deeper appreciation of how vital and essential the deep experiences of pain in my life had been. I appreciated, at a deeper level, the words of Jesus when he said that the only sign he would give this generation was 'the sign of Jonah; through the process of entering into the belly of the whale there was the promise of a new life'.

It is not only women who feel abandoned and it is not only men who have affairs! This is certainly reflected in our clinical experience and ratified by social commentators and the media. There is a problem that won't go away unless we address it. Men need to be able to speak and also to be heard. There has to be another way through. I know it is no longer acceptable for us, as women and mothers of sons, to hit out in anger at the male. Of course that reaction is understandable when women have felt hurt, neglected and abused at many levels, but at the end of the day it is an indulgence of the ego that we can ill afford and is an insult to our own soul and the integrity of who we really are. And besides, nobody ever wins a war.

We need to listen to statistics which tell us that 'the greatest cause of death in males between 16 and 60 is suicide', because something profoundly urgent is being said. If we don't, we will listen to our own wailing at the graves of our sons. Males and females have to find new eyes and ears to see and hear what our normal eyes and ears cannot. Perhaps our combined wounding and pain may be offering training in compassion and empathy for us to find a joint road home, via our soul-making, to each other as well as to ourselves.

Summary

- Both men and women experience hormonal change, but in men it is not so dramatic.
- Women's lack of sexual desire at midlife is often put down by men to hormonal changes. While this may be part of the problem, their relationship with their partner is often a contributing factor.
- Women at midlife need to be heard by their partner: they need to talk about the changes that are happening to them.
- Men may need professional help in dealing with their partners' crises and working through their own.
- Being abandoned by their partner is one of the greatest hurts for women at midlife, but it can also be an opportunity for profound change in each of them and between them.

23

Growing your relationship

In this birth you will discover all blessing
But neglect this birth and you neglect
all blessing. Tend only to this birth
in you and you will find there
all goodness and all consolation,
all delight, all being and
all truth.

Meister Eckhart (c. 1260–c. 1327)

I can still vividly remember the afternoon over five years ago when the phone rang and these words pierced me like a gigantic spear: 'They say I have ovarian cancer.' It was my close and much loved friend of twenty years on her way out of the doctor's surgery. As I raced over to see her, my thoughts got jammed in a paralysis of panic, a bit like a crowd running to get out of a burning building. How could this happen to someone so young, strong and vital with so much living still to be done? There must be a terrible mistake. The doctors have got it all wrong. God has got it wrong. I have got it wrong.

It took Jeanette fifteen months of fight, denial, struggle and grief punctuated with hilarity, ridiculous fun and wonderful friendship before she surrendered to her cancer. When she finally let go she felt her aloneness and her abandonment, the loss of her daughters, her family,

her house and garden, her friends and her life. She then began to appreciate the beauty in nature, the sound of a bird, the smell of a flower,
but most of all she began to appreciate *love*. Love for and from her two
daughters, her family and her friends, and life around her in all its manifestations. This love increasingly became gently interspersed with periods
of acceptance and peace. When Jeanette finally died I think she was
ready. I hope she thought so. Her process mirrored so much of my own
emotional surrender to reality that happened simultaneously. I was
letting go of old meanings I had given to my place in the world and the
roles I had played to support me in that place.

After the death of my mother and grandmother when I was just
thirteen, I compensated for this by making sure everyone loved me,
needed me and ultimately would never leave me. I became an absolute
master at reading people. If someone wanted a 'bright and breezy' I
would be there; if they needed a 'deep and meaningful' they could
count on me. In fact, I could give people what they wanted before they
even knew they wanted it. It became painfully clear I had spent my
adolescence and a good part of adulthood mentally on guard and at the
ready to advance my mission to be loved.

When Jeanette died I realised that I was battle fatigued. The burden
and emotional expenditure that goes with this degree of being needed
was too high a price to pay. I can't say I stopped caring what people said
or thought of me, but their opinion certainly lost its ultimate place of
importance. For a while it felt quite strange walking into a room full of
people and not having my radar antenna searching the room for positive and negative vibes. Or not spending hours on the telephone in
what felt like directing traffic in the relationships around me – warding
off danger or directing opportunity.

There is a parallel for women at midlife. Often we have invested so
many years in the lives of our children so that they will be loved,
respected and successful people that we sacrifice what *we* would like or
desire for what is best for *them*. We have supported our partners in their
careers and successes so that they will be good providers for our families.

We have built an emotional bunker for our tribe from which we pro-tect, defend and provide for their wellbeing. Then suddenly we find that our finely honed instinctual skills are no longer needed. I often hear men speaking of a similar process for them. Probably from before marriage, but certainly through the early years of establishing home and family, the man's primary focus is on providing. That is the way he cares for and expresses his love for his family. He receives recognition, validation and self-worth from being out there working hard. Then when he is 50 he turns around to spend well-earned time with his family. To his surprise, he finds he is with a group of strangers or that they have all gone. And this coincides with his wife's situation.

With family off her hands, she now spends time out of the home doing the things she has had on hold for a number of years. It seems a cruel irony that just when a man is ready to 'come home' the woman is probably ready to 'leave home'. I don't necessarily mean she wants to leave the marriage, although this can happen. Biologically and emo-tionally she has a reserve of energy that needs productive expression for her own wellbeing and for the good of the wider community. In primitive societies she would be welcomed into the circle of tribal elders where her accumulated wisdom would be both valued and employed.

Relationship is important at midlife. I always feel sad when relation-ships end for people at this time of their lives. It seems such a waste. All the years of hard work and the richness of shared joy and pain, lost. All the hopes and dreams of a lifetime, shattered. But it is at this time that prior years of neglect, unspoken hurt and resentment, and lack of understanding or appreciation, become like a boil that bursts.

This is a very painful and often messy time for a couple and their family and friends. Here are some symptoms that I am sure you know well, either from friends' or your own experience:

- She leaves because the love has just gone, buried under years of hurt and not being heard.

- He leaves for another women (possibly younger) because he feels that no matter what he does, she is never happy.
- He feels unseen and unappreciated by his partner of many years.

The only passions left in the relationship are anger and contempt.

Remember that a woman's most important sexual organ is her brain. If she doesn't feel loved, cared for or listened to in any other place but the bedroom, there will certainly be no sex. Not necessarily as a payback, nor because desire is absent, but because there is no motivation in her to try. A man, on the other hand, certainly needs sex, but often the reason he seeks out a younger woman is not just the 'sexy old man' stereotype, it is more likely that a younger woman has not been soured by the accumulation of hurt and disappointment that his wife has experienced. She is more likely to look up to and appreciate him with a new freshness, not the cynical criticism of years of unexpressed feelings.

I implore you. There is certainly a way through, but do not put it off and say, 'It doesn't matter, we'll get over it.' If you are reading this and recognise yourself, take this as your call to action. Even if you have a good relationship, there is always room for more depth and meaning no matter who you are. A partnership that is close, fun and enjoyable – a true sharing of mind, body and spirit – is worth time and effort. So why not try the following:

- Make a special appointment with your partner and say you need about one hour of uninterrupted time. Set the scene by explaining to him that he doesn't have to do or say anything and you would like him to be silent until you finish.
- Start by telling him three things you appreciate about him (e.g. that he has been a good provider, the way he has loved the children etc.).
- Make sure that you talk about yourself and your feelings not about his behaviour. In other words, make 'I' statements, not 'you' statements.

- Tell him about your dreams and longings, and then about the feelings inside that block you from bringing these dreams to fruition.
- If you are holding any hurt or resentment that is stopping you from feeling close to your partner, tell him about it. It is only then that you can let those hurts go. (Make sure you don't blame or criticise.)
- When you have completely finished, ask him if he would like to respond to anything you have said. He may want to think about it and respond later.
- Thank him for listening to you.

If you feel you need professional help, don't wait until the relationship is dead before you do something. Most treasured gifts in life are not just handed to us; we have to work for them. My own relationship of 22 years is no exception to this golden rule of life.

When Donatus and I got together I was just out of a failed marriage with three children aged nine, seven and five years. My new husband had spent the previous fifteen years living as a celibate priest in a monastery. Few, if any, gave us much of a chance. In fact, the odds of us making it for even one year were slim. Can you imagine the challenges we faced? For a start, Donatus felt that he knew next to nothing about women. The fact that he had no sisters and had entered an all-male Catholic seminary at the tender age of fifteen did little to help. And he suddenly found himself with what he felt were two powerful women, my daughter and myself, on his hands. It wasn't easy for any of us, and it really was a case of sink or swim. Swim we did, although sometimes it felt more like deep sea diving. I certainly had a number of issues from my childhood concerning abandonment that needed to be healed if my relationship with Donatus were to have a chance. I saw a therapist weekly for some months and later attended a group to help with my fear of being abandoned and my lack of self-worth. We faced painful issues. We learned to tell each other the truth no matter how difficult, learned to listen to each other and, perhaps most of all, we prayed and asked for help. The hard work has paid off and I feel very blessed and grateful for our relationship.

Midlife heralds a new stage of your relationship, with sexual, emotional and physical changes.

One of the greatest gifts motherhood gives is the absolute demand to look beyond the self: to become less self-centred in order to care for the other. It doesn't really matter how you feel. If the baby cries in the middle of the night you get up and tend the baby. Motherhood is a wonderful training ground, an initiate's school for *otherness consciousness*. Again, at midlife, our happiness depends on our ability to be aware of this 'otherness' around the birth of a new phase of our lives. I know that this thinking does not always find favour with the feminist in me or my friends, but I ask myself: 'Do I want to be right or do I want to be happy?'

As we learn from self psychology, mirroring is essential to the early development of the self. By focusing on her baby and mirroring its reality (e.g. smiling when baby smiles, making the same sound as the baby, looking sad when baby cries), the mother in fact plays a vital role in bringing to birth the baby's self. The woman is helped to develop these new muscles by the 'cuddle' hormone, oxytocin, which helps her to bond and stretch for her baby. Through this mirroring and stretching, the mother becomes more fully a woman and more grounded in the richness of her being. As many of you would have experienced, our lives have been enriched because we have had a part to play in the 'birthing' of our children.

This fertile and very practical concept of growth and transformation, in and through relationship, is underpinned by the seminal work of philosopher Martin Buber who, in his classic work, *I and Thou*, talks about how there is no 'I' without a 'You': 'One should beware altogether of understanding a conversation with (the Other) ... as something apart from or above the everyday.'

When we view our primary relationships through this window, we see the 'other' as our invitation to connection, wholeness and communion with our soul, not as a demand or distraction. It beckons us to move beyond the constricted self we think we are, and to expand into a bigger self. If couples understand this larger context, my experience is that they find it an effective and practical way for them to experience more happiness, fun and meaning in their relationships.

The need for otherness consciousness is most often required around the area of sex in our midlife relationships. You cannot lose on the happiness scale if you learn to be generous. An immediate feeling response to an invitation to make love might be no. But before you jump in with a reaction, it might be wise to take a helicopter view of how you really want to feel about yourself as a person and about your partner. If you continually feed thoughts like 'I don't feel sexual anymore' or 'All he wants is just one thing' or 'He can't even touch me without wanting sex', then you are going to end up feeling used, resentful, angry and unhappy. The odds are, with this sort of thinking, you are not going to feel too good about yourself either. The most dominating thoughts of your mind will eventually reproduce themselves in physical reality. If you want to be a confident, happy, loving and spiritually nourished person, you will need to feed loving, grateful thoughts into your mind and focus on seeing yourself as the person you want to be.

By the age of 45 you have a vast experience of life from which to draw your knowledge and wisdom. You have moved through the *self-consciousness* of youth and the *identity fight* of the feminist era. Now is the time for the more generous permission and relaxed freedom of mature *self-awareness* that comes to fruition precisely through well-practised *otherness consciousness*. May I suggest you try the following each day for 30 days and watch the results.

Every morning think about the following to start building the person you want to be:

Happy	(three things you feel happy about)
Excited	(three things you feel excited about)
Proud	(three things or people you feel proud of)

Grateful	(three things you feel grateful for)
Enjoying	(three things you enjoy)
Loving	(three people you love and three who love you)

You can use the same things every day if you can't think of new ones. If you really want these feelings to be expressed in your life, write them down in an exercise book each day. Then follow this by writing a description of the person you want to be. Watch what happens!

Summary

- Relationship is extremely important to us at midlife, yet it may be a time when husband and wife, or partners, become more estranged, and even break up.
- With courage to let go of old patterns of relating and willingness to feel uncomfortable while trying something new, midlife can be the time to create space for trusting friendship to grow and love to deepen.
- Issues that have not been addressed and resentments that have been pushed aside are most likely to present at midlife. Love can continue to flow, and in fact deepen, if couples are willing to work at it. The rewards are enormous.
- Relationship at midlife can be a rich and fruitful arena for spiritual deepening and growth.
- There are times when we need a coach or professional help. Don't wait till it is too late.

Part 4

Attitudinal change to menopause

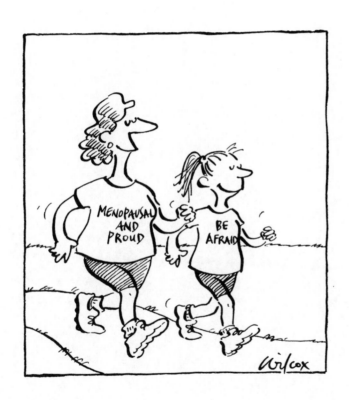

Attitudinal change to your ... menopause

24

Mum, have you got your patch on?

Out of the mouths of babes and sucklings hast thou ordained strength.

Psalm 8, Verse 2

'Mum, have you got your patch on?' was a question asked of a menopausal older mother by her six-year-old daughter. Nothing is hidden these days, thank goodness. The old days of secrets and lies are giving way as young girls deal very directly with the facts of life, beginnings and endings, and everything that happens in between.

Menarche, the beginning of menstruation, should be no surprise today as it is part of the school curriculum. My own story of nearly 60 years ago illustrates well the difference between then and now. Just before my 12th birthday (I should really say 'our' birthday as I have a twin sister, but she is half an hour younger and, as usual, I was ahead of her), I woke in the middle of the night wet and uncomfortable. I went out to the toilet on the back verandah (we were lucky, for many Australian families the toilet was at the end of the backyard and called 'the dunny'). I was distressed and very surprised to find that I was bleeding. But bleeding from where? I can still remember the fear that I was bleeding to death and I did not know why. I had had nosebleeds before but that was from the other end. I had no idea *whatsoever* of my anatomy 'down there'. When my mother found me at 6 am, pale and weepy, she was hardly reassuring and she certainly did not explain the mystery to me. In fact she was so shame-faced herself that there were no questions I could ask. From that time on I thought of periods as disgusting and a great nuisance. The war between my hormones and me had begun! I have talked about this war in Chapter 8.

Older women, like myself, remember when there were no such things as disposable tampons or pads. The other part of my own menstrual nightmare was that we had four women in our household and we shared squares of old sheets torn up and used with belts and safety pins to cope with the dreaded, and to my mind cursed, monthly flow. These rags were soaked in a bucket and then boiled up in the copper. It was all totally disgusting. I understand now how the lack of information and initiation scarred (and scared) me emotionally.

In New Guinea ... a woman who has permanently ceased menstruation is ... accorded status, which she did not have in her premenopausal phase of life.

Nowadays, most young women are prepared for their first period and are encouraged to view the onset of menstruation with some pride and celebration. But more could be done. In ancient cultures there were suitable ceremonies for young women, as well as young men, at puberty. There was also recognition of the ending of menstruation in many cultures.

In New Guinea, for example, a woman who has permanently ceased menstruation is able to sit with the men at meetings. She is accorded status, which she did not have in her premenopausal phase of life. Interestingly, village women in New Guinea do not have sanitary pads. The flow is seldom very heavy and lasts only one or two days. Sometimes they use balls of grass to stem the flow, but usually they just squat in the 'haus blud' (blood house), which also is the 'haus pig'. (Pigs are more valuable than women in the highlands society so are protected and sheltered.) Women have to be away from the men at this time because the menstrual flow is considered poisonous to men!

In fact, as discussed earlier, menstruation is not common in the 'primitive' woman. She is either pregnant or fully breastfeeding for most of her reproductive life, providing that she survives the dangers of childbirth, and has fewer than 50 periods in all. On the other hand, the modern woman squeezes childbearing into two to five years and has about 40 years of monthly cycles and thus about 400 menstrual periods in a lifetime. 'Primitive' women do not suffer from the dysfunctional type of bleeding that has become so common in our own society as menstrual cycles become unbalanced in the lead-up to menopause.

For some women now reaching menopause, there is still a veil of silence behind which their mothers have retreated. Many women have expressed regret and anger that their mothers could not share their experiences about this other watershed in their lives.

'I had no prior warning or training', said Rita. 'My mother refused to speak about anything pertaining to her own menstrual cycle or sex. At menopause she closed up even more. I do remember that she became housebound and was always fanning herself. I was 25 then and had already left home. My father told me to go carefully around her because "she is easily upset you know". Well, I *didn't* know! I would have liked to know what was happening for her and what she was feeling, but there was nothing – just this wall of silence.'

For many women menopause was not named and it was not to be spoken about. I asked my elderly aunt recently about her experiences. 'How long does menopause last?' I asked her. 'Menopause is ten years coming and ten years going,' said my aunt cheerfully. This did not cheer me up at all.

Rita is now 47 and is having an early menopause. She was a career woman and married late. She had her first daughter when she was 39, then adopted a baby two years later. It was this little girl, now aged six, who asked her the memorable question that is the title for this chapter: 'Mum, have you got your patch on?' These girls at their tender ages are very aware of Rita's ups and downs. Unlike her own mother who shared nothing with her, Rita has decided to talk to her own girls. Perhaps they are too young to fully appreciate what is happening, but they certainly do know when Mum's hormones are up or down.

Rita has some questions about her menopausal phase. At times she finds it hard to maintain the control that has got her this far, first as a career woman and now combining career and motherhood, at this major crossroads in her life: menopause. There is a family history of mental breakdown, which worries her. She is concerned that she may also be prone to breakdown and that her husband could leave her if this happened. She confided to me that she knows that she could not cope with the girls alone if this happened.

Rita is experiencing some of the pitfalls of late motherhood. Age does produce some physical limitations, but the emotional changes that occur as the biological clock winds down are the significant challenges, and these have brought many women to their knees. Women in their late forties and early fifties are meant to be *grandmothers* of small children, not mothers. They need to be able to give the demanding ones back to a younger mother!

Rita is on HRT. It has relieved the physical symptoms like hot flushes and helped her to keep on a more even keel emotionally. I do not think alternative therapies would be enough here. She needs all the help she can get. The patch is her badge. I can't imagine her small daughter enquiring if she has taken her phytoestrogen (the plant or 'natural' estrogens, which are not a substitute for the real thing).

This chapter illustrates the interaction of the mind and emotions with hormones. Women with conflicting responsibilities, such as young children and career, can face quite a watershed if the ups and downs of menopause are added to these. HRT can certainly save the day for some. And women's openness with their partner and children about menopause is another step in the right direction.

Summary

- The veil of silence has been removed from the onset of menstruation, which is now generally understood by girls and celebrated.
- Increasingly, too, women are better able to discuss menopause with their partner and children, although there is still a long way to go.
- HRT has been helpful for some women in stabilising the physical and emotional symptoms of this stage in their lives so that it no longer has to be endured in silence and pain.

25

Where have all the grandmas gone?

Don't wait for light to appear at the end of the tunnel, stride down there ... and light the bloody thing yourself.

Sara Henderson, author

It seems that age is no longer an excuse for anything. The Nike slogan 'Just do it' has been taken up enthusiastically by young sportswomen and men but also by grandmas! The sky's the limit. Grandmas nowadays climb mountains, swim the English Channel, learn to fly, complete PhDs, have another baby (well, in Italy or France, at any rate), enter politics, become prime minister.

A verse, author unknown, which always strikes a chord with older women we talk to in groups, has the same theme:

In the dim and distant past
When life's tempo wasn't fast,
Grandma used to rock and knit,
Crochet, tat and babysit.
When the kids were in a jam,

They could always call on 'Gran'.
In that day of gracious living,
Grandma was the gal for giving.
But, today she's in the gym,
Exercising to keep slim,
She's off touring with the bunch,
Or taking clients out to lunch.
Going north to ski or curl,
All her days are in a whirl.
Nothing seems to stop or block her,
Now that grandma's off her rocker.

Grandmothers have an important, though changing, role in our society. Some are too busy for the role; others complain that there is no role for them anymore!

Judy is now 70 and is 20 years past menopause. She took HRT for five years but no longer needs it. Her bone density is excellent. She has no heart attack risks.

Her husband died fifteen years ago. Her children were all independent at an early age, and have their own families. Every second year she and a friend, also a postmenopausal grandma, go to some out of the way place. They trek, they climb mountains, and they canoe. Last year they went bungee jumping in New Zealand. Her children have to ask well in advance if they want any babysitting done!

Judy's own mother lived a sheltered life, did not drive a car and never travelled further than a hundred miles from her hometown. She died a frail old woman at 75, after fracturing her hip because of osteoporosis. Judy, on the other hand, is a modern grandmother who is seizing opportunities at this stage of her life. She herself has flown the nest.

Pauline, aged 54, feels redundant because her daughter-in-law allows her little time with her two grandchildren. She has only one son. She used to be close to him, but now she is feeling pushed away by his wife. 'It's a pity to waste grandmothers', she said to me sadly. She has time on her hands these days. She does not work and her husband is not yet retired. She would love to babysit her grandchildren. When her son brings them to visit her it takes time for them to settle and be comfortable with her.

The grandmother role has changed in the last twenty years, in barely a generation.

Many women in their sixties are still waiting to be grandmothers as their children in their late thirties continue to ignore the biological clock. For some there will be no grandchildren. Women's sexual freedom, thanks largely to the Pill, has made childbearing and even marriage optional. Yes, it is a pity to waste grandmothers, but perhaps Pauline and others like her can find a way to use this energy and fill this longing.

'The idea of old age is also changing ... Women in their sixties and seventies do not get old. Instead we enter an active and satisfying "third age" ...'

'The idea of old age is also changing', says Sheila Kitzinger (of natural childbirth fame). 'Women in their sixties and seventies do not get old. Instead we enter an active and satisfying "third age" and after that, at eighty, a happy and contented "fourth age".' Grandmothers and non-grandmothers have an average life expectancy nowadays of 85. Physical and mental health is needed so that this fourth age can be happy and also healthy.

Although medicalisation of the menopause has been viewed by some natural therapists as an unwarranted takeover bid by doctors and pharmaceutical companies, there is no doubt that the catch cry 'feminine forever' and the introduction of HRT in the sixties has led to improved health promotion programs for women. Again, I stress that I am *not* advocating HRT for all, but I do advocate, for all women, a proper assessment at this stage of life. Grandmothers these days have benefits that their own grandmothers did not. Women, on average, live longer than men. Most women I know have the ability to bear emotional stress and to cope with loss better than men do. 'A woman is like a teabag', said Nancy Reagan, 'You can't tell how strong she is until you put her in hot water.'

Some grandmothers are concerned about their adult children (usually male) who don't leave home, but take over the father/husband role.

Among a group of women with whom I was discussing the changing role of grandmothers, some became very vocal when they started to consider their own predicament. Divorced or widowed after many years of marriage, they had sons who refused to leave home and had taken over a patriarchal role in the household. These sons were adults, but in some ways still children, who had taken over the role of husband, making decisions and generally living their lives with little reference to their mother's wants or needs. The mothers continued to do all the washing and to cook the meals. They paid most of the household bills. They would like to have grandchildren but their sons do not want to commit to a family of their own.

Serena says that her 30-year-old son refuses to leave home because he thinks *she* is not capable of living alone. He treats her with little respect. Serena says, 'Coming of age for boys is not 21 but 30. We've got them until then and often beyond. The girls leave home and get married and/ or make their own household and have children but the boys stay on as lords of the manor.'

Serena feels that many young people, and boys in particular, are afraid to commit to marriage especially if the marriage of the parents failed. Serena and her son snap at each other. It is not an easy situation for her, but he persists in staying.

Joy's husband died a year ago. She is still grieving. Her son has moved back home and taken over the house. He has not only taken over the role of his father but also his mannerisms! This is not what she wants and she asks, 'What possesses these children to feel that we need a man about the house, a pseudo-husband?'

Some mothers go on rescuing their sons; even when the children do move out they buy them cars, refrigerators and so on. They still do their washing and ironing. Some of the sons are perpetual students unprepared to go out and earn a living or take on responsibility. They are prepared to earn less money and have more leisure. Many do not want the sort of career or work ethic that their fathers had.

As this group of women continued to discuss the changing role of grandmothers other issues arose. It was not just the boys or young men that had their mothers puzzled. Some grandmothers felt trapped; others felt free.

Hormones have very little to do with these feelings, but there is no doubt that HRT for some women improves quality as well as quantity of life. Now that daughters are choosing to delay having children, their mothers have to wait longer to become grandmothers so HRT can be helpful in keeping these women fit for the grandmother role. For some of them, however, this new wellness makes them so independent that they are not much available to fulfil this role!

I believe that it is now time to ask also, 'Where have all the grandpas gone?'

Far too many of them have succumbed to heart attacks and strokes. Even in these days of being aware of the dangers of smoking and high cholesterol, many of them retire and drop dead, leaving an excess of grandmas doing their own thing. I believe that men also should have a complete assessment at middle age of their physical mental and emotional wellbeing. Unfortunately, clinics for this purpose are rare in this country.

Summary

- The grandmother role has changed considerably in the last twenty years.
- Some grandmothers may still provide support to their sons and daughters and their grandchildren, but they may also live very fulfilling separate lives themselves.
- Some regret the lack of involvement with grandchildren, both for themselves and for their grandchildren, as they know how important grandparents are in the lives of grandchildren.
- Others are faced with the problem of sons, in particular, living at home till their thirties and taking on the role of the husband who has died or is divorced from their mother.
- Yet others do not become grandmothers till their sixties or seventies, if at all, with both men and women delaying having children until their late thirties.

Part 5

Healing ways

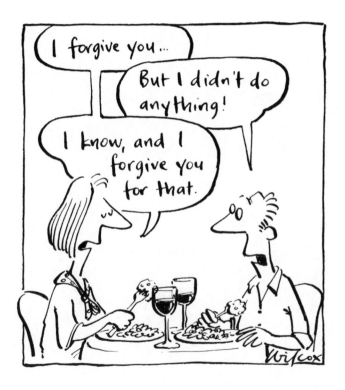

26

Forgiveness –
the healing balm and the key to happiness

The holiest place on earth is where an ancient hatred becomes a present love.

A Course in Miracles

What could you want that forgiveness cannot give?
*   Do you want peace? Forgiveness offers it. Do you want happiness, a quiet mind,*
a certainty of purpose and a sense of worth and beauty that transcends the world?
Do you want care and safety and the warmth of sure protection always? Do you
want a quietness that cannot be disturbed, a gentleness that never can be hurt, a
deep abiding comfort and a rest so perfect it can never be upset? All this, forgiveness
offers you and more.

A Course in Miracles

Forgiveness is one of those loaded words, like God. Sadly, because of this, the profound and treasured gifts that forgiveness bears are often pushed away, passed over or rejected out of hand. We often come across people who have been inoculated against it from a past bad religious experience, or who have seen friends or acquaintances profess a pseudo-forgiveness that has turned them off forever.

One of the most common misconceptions is that forgiveness con-
dones hurtful, harmful negative behaviour. If we forgive, it is seen as
'letting them off the hook'. This is not true; justice still needs to be done
– if possible, justice that will restore hope, not just punitive justice. The
only person you are 'letting off the hook' is you. By releasing the anger,
hate and vengeance you are making a powerful decision to no longer
suffer, a decision to heal your heart and mind. Another misconception
is that to forgive means that we have to deny our feelings and pretend
that what we see with our eyes or feel inside us is not really happening.
This is not true. There are unhealthy consequences for people who deny
their feelings.

Kate was a good-looking, 48-year-old executive accountant, divorced,
with two adult children. She said she had a 'job from heaven' in an
industry she loved and felt passionate about. She said, 'So why do I
want to toss it all away? I am tired, depressed and just don't want to get
up in the morning.' Her 24-year-old daughter was expecting her first
child and, in Kate's own words, 'I should be the happiest person alive!'

Kate went on to say how different her daughter's first pregnancy was
to her own. Kate had fallen pregnant at sixteen and had been forced by
her parents to go interstate to give birth and have the baby adopted out.
As life would have it, her baby boy was stillborn.

As she recalled the story she began to cry, then sob, saying that at
the time she was relieved and just wanted to get on with her life and
leave the tragic events behind her. However, she had never grieved the
loss of her baby or felt the pain and anger at her parents' rejection and
lack of support. I had her write a letter to her 'lost baby' and she
decided to name him David. In a few months, after experiencing all the
feelings that had been buried for so long, Kate was beginning to feel her
old happy self. Ultimately, Kate's forgiveness of herself and her parents
was a gift of love to herself.

Women at midlife are often still carrying pain, guilt and blame from terminations of pregnancy that they had years before. Another huge issue is resentment held towards husbands for not being there for them around the birth of their baby. Forgiveness holds the key to release for both these groups of women.

A further misconception is that to forgive makes us weak and unprotected. We feel that we are giving others the green light to hurt us again. If we forgive, it somehow makes them right and us wrong. For some strange reason we hold the belief that anger is stronger than the power of love. Sometimes, when we feel hurt, the voice inside comes from a place of fear. When we don't forgive we are the ones who suffer and lose our sense of peace.

Love is the strongest source of power in the world. No matter how much we are hurting, somewhere deep inside there is always a choice. Do I want to be right or do I want to be happy? I see women in their roles of mothers and lovers being in a place of power and influence in a world that needs to be shown that love really is stronger than fear. The following story, written by Don Goewey, the director of the Centre for Attitudinal Healing in Sausalito, USA, is from his book *Fishing for Fallen Light*. Goewey went to Bosnia with a group of volunteers in response to a request from three women – Maja, Melita and Vesna. They asked for help to heal the hatred in the hearts of their people raped and torn apart by war. He writes:

Together with a few others, these three women rent a house and make it cosy for the broken-hearted pilgrims. This house is available for everyone. There is no discrimination. Everyone touched by war is welcome.

One day some people at this little house suggest a simple proposition: 'Let's form a group and talk.' Serbs, Muslims, Croats, everyone and anyone. A deep suspicion and chill of fear greets this proposal. It quickly raises Cain among the men. The world in which this war is waging has cut a line into their minds, a line they think they cannot cross.

In the back of the room a woman stands to talk. She adjusts her heavy mass and leans into her cane and says, 'I am from Sarajevo. A Muslim. The Serbs killed my father and took away my husband. I encouraged in my boys this hatred that is killing us. I sent them off to fight. Can you believe it? I thought that hatred in their hearts would make them strong and keep them safe.'

She shakes her head and for a time her eyes grow dim. Then she continues:

'They were killed in combat not much more than a month apart. They came back home to me in canvas bags. I tell you this: **I was the one who killed my sons. Not the Serbs. I killed them with my hatred.** And until my dying day I will say to every mother everywhere I go, teach your children love. Even for their enemy. It's hatred that will kill them.'

For me this is not a story about a woman in Bosnia. It is a story about me. When I hear it I feel a personal invitation to let go of the anger and separation in my heart, not just for my sake but also for the sake of my children and grandchildren. It's a powerful story that speaks to my heart. It is particularly relevant now in a world that has changed since the events of September 11, 2001. I listen to people here in Australia who are living their lives in a rubble heap of fear and uncertainty in the midst of their own family. I can only imagine what it must be like for those in the USA, Afghanistan and Iraq.

This Muslim woman's plea puts the ball right back in my court. I may feel impotent in changing the opinion of world leaders but I can do something about the divisions inside my own heart. I know I have a terrorist inside me that, when hurt, wants to lash out and blame others. I hear this story as an invitation to let go of old pain and resentment. One thought leads to another and then another and collectively they are a force for good. So it's not just for my own inner peace, but the peace of the world, that I feel empowered to do something instead of worry.

Another misconception about forgiveness is that, if you forgive, you will have to do things you don't want to do, such as becoming 'best friends' with your ex-husband or spending time with a person that has been hurtful. This is not true. You are not being asked to have warm feelings or to like this person. You are being asked to see this person you hate or feel so angry towards, no matter what he or she has done, as a human being. You may not be able to feel love, but for the sake of your own freedom you can step back and allow life, or God, to love this person. You can step back and allow love to find a way.

One of the most painful things you can do to yourself is to hold another person out of your heart. One of the key words around forgiveness is *willingness*. Sometimes it is almost impossible to imagine what it would be like to forgive a certain person in your life. It is just too hard to even contemplate. All that is required to start the process is a little willingness. I once had a woman say to me that she 'wanted to want' to forgive her father for his abuse towards her. I assured her that that was all she needed for the melting of the hurt and pain to begin. For her own happiness and peace of mind she wanted to let go of the angry, painful thoughts she was holding towards him. Slowly she began to withdraw the angry negative thoughts and, after some time, she was able to see her father surrounded by love. She couldn't feel a personal love for him, but she could manage to see him surrounded by love. This was a great breakthrough for her healing and future happiness.

Why forgive? Forgiveness is the key to happiness; it releases us from a painful past. The roots of our pain are like a gnarled old tree stump that's buried deep down inside. No wonder it hurts! Forgiveness unties the tangled mess and eventually helps us let go of the anger, hurt and blame that are causing the pain and distress.

When you are upset you always focus on what you don't want. When you are feeling down or hurt by someone, do you find yourself getting out the 'logbook' and remembering all the other times this person has hurt you in the past, and loading shovels full of fuel onto the furnace of hurt and pain to justify your stand? I know I have. But does it get you what you want? Does it make you or anyone else happier or safer, more joyful or peaceful?

You can't stop the initial feeling but you can, with some practice, stop fuelling the fire of justification and unhappiness. It helps to remember that you have a choice: you don't have to be a victim. Honour the hurt feelings, and then in the name of your own freedom and kindness to yourself, be willing to release them. The brain doesn't understand negative commands. What you focus on is what you get, so it helps to say what you want and what you are willing to do to get it. Telling your brain you are willing to do whatever it takes to be happy and peaceful puts your feet on the road of forgiveness and, ultimately, peace and happiness. Forgiveness stops the past from inevitably being repeated in the future. It means living in the present without the shadows of the past.

Most of us are careful about ingesting dangerous fumes or drugs because we are aware of the detrimental side effects. Yet we are not nearly so careful about the toxic thoughts we allow to live 'rent free' in our head. Our minds are very good computers and what we program in has enormous consequences on our feelings, our bodies and our relationships. It is certainly possible to reprogram our negative thoughts. Sometimes we are carrying things around in our head and we don't even know this. My dad, who died two years ago, was a pretty tough cop as I was growing up, a real man's man. When he was in his sixties he started to get palpitations in his chest and was quite a stress-prone, grumpy old man. Some years later, much to my surprise as well as his, he attended one of the 'Forgiveness Seminars' that my husband and I were running at the time: 'Just to take a look at this *stuff* you're always rabbiting on about.' He said nothing after the seminar. When I asked him if he had liked it he said he supposed it was okay for some people. A week later he called in to see us one late afternoon saying, 'You know that stuff you do really works!' When I asked him how he came to that conclusion he told me what had happened.

He was travelling down a busy highway towards the university where he swam every day; he was running behind schedule and, of course, in a hurry. As he approached a busy intersection he just missed the green light and was stuck for some time waiting for the red light to change. He said his heart was thumping, he felt angry and uptight, and he was gripping the steering wheel 'like I was in a bloody car rally'. He then related how he happened to notice that he was thinking of an old superintendent who had wrongly accused him when he was a young cop and how angry he was when he recalled feeling betrayed by this man. Then he began to laugh and give himself a talking to: 'Well, I'm a silly old fool. Here I am thousands of miles away and 50 years down the track. That old beggar I'm thinking about is probably dead and buried.' He said he thought to himself, 'Well, I can rest assured he is not thinking about me; the only person whose gut is in an uproar is mine.' In that moment he let go of the past and said to himself: 'Just let that silly old fool rest in peace!'

After discovering how effective had been this letting go of old feelings and reactions my father then started a whole process of letting go of many other painful things in his past. He looked for a nice thing to say about every person he met and volunteered his time to be of service at the Centre of Attitudinal Healing where he made many new friends. For the last 15 years of my father's life he was a very happy, loving man surrounded by family and friends who loved him.

An exercise in forgiveness

- Sit in a chair and think of a person you are feeling angry towards.
- Let all the feelings you have about this person flood into you.
- How does your body feel?
- Make a list of all the feelings, both physical and emotional.

You now have the beginnings of a list of feelings you are carrying around 'rent free' in your head. Why would you want to poison yourself with all that toxicity? As an act of loving kindness to yourself, be willing to let these feelings go – to forgive.

I am often asked how long it takes to forgive. My friend and teacher, Dr Jerry Jampolsky, says:

It is never too early to forgive.
It is also never too late to forgive.
Forgiveness takes as long as you believe it will take.
If you believe it will never happen.
It will never happen.
If you believe it will take six months.
It will take six months.
If you believe it will take but a second
That's all that it will take.

Summary

- Forgiveness does not condone harmful, hurtful behaviour. Non-punitive justice still needs to be done.
- Forgiveness only asks that you see the person who has wounded you as a human being in all his or her frailty.
- Forgiveness does not mean denying your negative feelings towards another; that is unhealthy. You need to honour your hurt feelings and then release them.
- By letting go of negative feelings and acting through love, not anger or fear, the person you are forgiving is you.
- All you need is a willingness to forgive.

27

Love finds a way

A man shall leave his mother and a woman leave her home
So they can travel on, and the two shall be as one.

'The Wedding Song'

What you offer to others you experience within yourself. What you see in others you strengthen in yourself. When you approach life fearfully, you actually install the 'triggers' in your brain, which you then blame others for pulling. This is painfully evident in our relationships with our adolescent children. I often have parents coming to me at the 'end of the road' in total fear, anger and desperation, not knowing what to do with their son or daughter. The fear is particularly acute when the child is involved in illicit drug taking.

I have a lot of compassion and empathy for these parents. I too felt my guts ripping apart in impotent fear, when one of our children became involved in the drug scene. Craig was 16 when it all began. By the time he was 17 he had moved out of home into a shared house, but to all intents and purposes he was somewhere out there 'living on the street'. We lived in what seemed like a constant state of alert and fear. We felt guilty. We blamed him and ourselves. We felt that he was blaming us. We tried 'strong arm' control tactics. We tried every single psychological skill and/or manipulation that we or any of our colleagues could come up with. We thought at one stage of getting private detectives to follow him so that we had some idea of what he was doing. But of course none of this worked. The only thing we succeeded in doing was to alienate Craig even further and drive ourselves into despair. The one thing left for us was prayer. Not that we hadn't been praying already, but now we were stripped bare with nothing else to do and nowhere else to turn.

Sooner or later in life many of us seem to be given the opportunity … to surrender to a greater freedom.

Sometimes in the middle of the night I would awake to the sound of police sirens somewhere in the distance. In those dark, haunted hours fear and panic are never far away in the corridors of the mind.

I am trying to describe the inner struggle that often precedes surrender into a deeper and fuller freedom. Sooner or later in life many of us seem to be given the opportunity to confront that basic struggle within, a chance to surrender to a greater freedom. This was certainly such a time for me. We don't seem to realise that there is no basis for the struggle, and that we (and our loved ones) are truly safe in the arms of love, no matter what happens. For me, that surrender was a process spread out over many years, but it came to a head at this time. Like most victories, it came with a struggle. Could I truly believe that, whatever the outcome, I would be saved by this power of love, which I believed in but sometimes forgot to trust. I knew first hand what it was like to have loved ones suddenly, tragically torn from me. I had experienced the horror of the 'knock at the door' bearing the unbearable when my mother and grandmother were killed. I was just thirteen at that time and had never been away from home until that weekend. So, of course, the panic and dread that this might happen again was almost more than I could contain.

Looking back on those harrowing nights, I realise that I had nowhere else to go. In a sense, I really had no viable choice but to surrender Craig and myself into a higher love and reality. Like a deer cornered with its back to the rock face and trapped by baying hounds, I had a reason, as well as desperation, to leap into a new freedom through surrender. I made a decision to use these times in the night as an opportunity. When I woke, rather than worry, I would see Craig surrounded by a 'portable safety zone' of grace and held in the arms of love. No matter where he was or what he was doing, I would send him love.

On occasions, he would call around to the house to see us. I would see nothing but the best in him. I would see how difficult it was for him to come and how brave he was. I refused the mind's invitation to put energy into his thin emaciated body or appearance. One day I went around to the house where he was staying, knocked on the door and asked if I could clean it. I was privileged that he still had enough trust to let me in. I cleaned the house and filled the fridge with food. I prayed for strength, and made a commitment to see the young people in the house as hurting inside and needing love and acceptance right where they were. I continued this every few weeks for some months – I am not sure how many. It was as many months as I needed. I found that, as I cleaned the house, it was my heart and soul that were cleaned of the arrogance and judgements I held about youth, drugs, and what I considered good and bad behaviour, and so much more. After all, I was a policeman's daughter, and the policeman inside my head went crazy with what I saw. But gradually and through the power of love I was cleansed as I cleaned.

My husband and I would spend time every morning and evening seeing him surrounded by *unconditional love*. Towards the end of this period I had a dream in which Craig was a baby at my breast. In the dream he briefly stopped feeding to give me a delighted milky smile. I continually used this image to see his delight and innocence and to feel just how very much I loved him. A short time after this, in the early hours of the morning, Craig came to the house and into our room and woke us very distressed. I held him and we all just cried. He moved back home soon after this, and then began the long healing and rehabilitating process inside us all. Today Craig is a man who has my profound respect and love. He is a human being of power, passion and integrity, with an enormous capacity for love. More than most men I know he has faced his shadow and the demons inside him and has, with the grace of God, come out the other side a very beautiful human being.

Forgiveness means seeing the light of God in everyone, regardless of their behaviour.

Practising the power of love

- See only the best in people.
- Become a 'love finder', rather than a 'fault finder'.
- See people surrounded with a light of love. Do this silently from your heart while driving, waiting forever for recorded messages on the telephone, or passing people on the street. Do it with people you feel close to and people you are having difficulty with.
- Celebrate your little victories. Affirm yourself when you have managed to do something that required effort. When you accomplish something say, 'I did it.' Then describe what you did.
- When someone does something that hurts you, be aware that you have a choice; you can see intentional acts of meanness, or mistakes from someone who is hurting inside and is giving a call for help.
- Begin each day being grateful for at least three things. Before closing your day make sure you have told each person in your household something you appreciate about them.

I see so much hurt, anger and confusion in families as children try to separate from the family. It is often very confusing. The child that the mother once had a strong bond with and who was a delight in her life suddenly becomes moody, secretive and angry. It doesn't help that the mother is probably going through menopause (just to add a bit more flavour to the soup). Dad is often 'thrown for a loop' as well. This can bring tension into the parents' relationship and the whole family can become embroiled in a very intense and distressing time. It really helps to know this is not happening because you are a bad parent or you have done something wrong. In fact, it often means you are a very good parent who has given your child enough security so that he or she can 'slam the door'.

In our present society, not only does the front door get slammed, but the child comes back through the window. The adolescent still living at home and needing the support of the family also needs to separate and is trying to do this. Only the very brave, courageous parent and child dare venture onto this precarious path. We are the first generation where there are children at home who need support while going through university or who cannot afford to leave home for other reasons. Yet these young ones have enough courage to want to walk their own path, to be independent. They want reassurance from us and they ask, 'Will you still love me, even if I don't live the life you have designed for me?'

One of the key developmental stages of our personality is the need to separate emotionally from our family as part of the journey into adulthood. In some cultures this transition is supported by a 'rite of passage' ceremony. There is usually some symbolic way in which the child leaves the mother to join 'the men' or 'the women' and leaves behind childhood to become an adult. This way the parent isn't left feeling a sense of guilt or failure, rather the parting is broadly accepted and respected. The community supports the child and the parent. Our youngest child, Meneesha, didn't wait until she was an adolescent to do this; in fact she started at about the age of five. One busy morning my husband was trying to hurry her up to get to preschool and told her she had to be in the car in two minutes or else! She wheeled on him and said; 'I am not a cat or a dog for you to talk to me like that; I'm a child and you shouldn't say that to children.'

From a tender age she had a keenly developed sense of self, which demanded its own integrity and respect. I think because she was born ten years after the other children who were ten, twelve and fourteen when she was born, there was enough emotional space for her. She was totally loved, not only by her two parents, but also by the other three children. This gave her a very strong sense of self, and it was from this position that she had enough security to be her own person from an early age.

This didn't just appear out of thin air. When Donatus and I got together the children were six, eight and ten years old. Following the upheaval and break-up of my first marriage and then the starting of a new relationship, the children were very insecure. I knew it was essential for me to do some things differently in my own life if these children were to have any sense of control and power over their own lives. At the same time I needed to convey to them how much I loved them and how very important they were to me. Because of my age (32) we really wanted to have a baby soon after we were married.

We knew it was important to include the three children in this process. When we asked them how they would feel about us having a baby they were adamant with a resounding 'NO'. We listened to them and decided to leave it until they were ready.

I knew in my bones that if this new family unit was to have a chance of working I had some serious letting go to do. There really had to be another way. The biggest thing I had to do was to forgive my ex-husband, the children's father, and myself for all the pain and bitterness that we inflicted on each other during our time together. For my children's sake and my own, I had to let go of the anger and resentment I was holding.

I started with a letter to myself, telling me how loved I was and why I needed and deserved to forgive and be forgiven. I told Patricia in the letter that I wanted to do this as an act of love for her. I then wrote a letter (not to send) to my ex-husband forgiving him and asking to be forgiven. I started to visualise a bridge of easy access back and forth between the children and him. Eventually I found the courage to phone him, and then down the track to meet for a cup of coffee. Ever so slowly, because we were both very frightened, the process continued. I will never forget, two years later, the look on the faces of the children when their Dad came to have an evening meal with us for the first time since we had split. *Love had found a way.*

Spearheaded by our eldest son, Mark, three years on from the time when we originally spoke to the children about a baby, we received an exuberant, overwhelmingly excited 'YES'. We had paved a way to make room for a baby. The pregnancy brought the whole family together in a new identity, shared focus and loving bond. This also brought Margaret Smith into our lives when I chose her as an obstetrician. I asked Margaret how she would feel if I brought the whole family to the prenatal visits so they could be included in the lead-up to the arrival of this new member of our family. To help the children feel fully included, providing it was medically safe, I wanted to have this baby at home. Meneesha was born at home with just Donatus, the children and a midwife present. Margaret arrived just fifteen minutes later. A week or so after this, Mark put a bumper sticker across his bedroom door proclaiming 'Home Is Where the Birth Is'. When we saw this we realised that we had not only birthed a new baby girl, but also a new family unit. This unit was going to be a place where the six of us would negotiate the joy, pain, sorrow and celebration of our unfolding lives and future.

The above story about identity raises a vitally important issue that I want to discuss, and that is *deadness* in a relationship. If you don't feel 'at home' when you are together, and you have to walk on eggshells around each other, it's quite probable that the rot set in early during your life together. This doesn't mean it's too late. It's quite likely that you didn't talk about things that you thought would cause trouble or that you ran around trying to 'please' rather than being yourself. Conflict was probably viewed as bad, and therefore avoided, because you didn't know how to deal with it.

When I see these things happening to a couple I ask them how they separated from their own families as adolescents. Did your family have the unspoken rule: 'Play by our rules and you will be loved.' The long-term price paid for 'being good' is feeling lost, living a life of quiet desperation. You become like a robot on a conveyor belt. You become a master of the game of pretence. This pretence stops you from ever

238 Is IT ME OR MY HORMONES?

feeling loved because there is always the hidden clause, 'If you really knew who I was you wouldn't love me.' This is a symptom of a child who has only known conditional love – 'play by the family rules or be rejected'.

Often the reason for our really deep distress as our children go through adolescent separation is the realisation that we didn't go through this separation for ourselves. As children we develop techniques for being safe, being loved, being significant, being cared for and so on. It is very difficult to let all this go in the name of being ourselves. Would the real me please stand up? Often we don't know who that is because there has been so much pretence, and resentment, guilt and depression can set in. Fear is the fiercest excluder, ceaselessly dividing. Love is the gatherer, forever including. It's never too late. There has to be, and there is, another way. All you need is a little willingness and love will find a way.

Forgiveness is the way through. Forgiveness is grace in action. Grace comes from within. It clears the clots of our constraints. When we welcome grace into our lives, blocks and grievances fall away, the veil lifts, and the heart opens.

Forgiveness means not excluding your love from anyone.

Freeing your heart to love

Here are some practical suggestions to soothe, heal and gently free your heart to love:

- Write letters (not to send) to yourself or your parents or significant others. Deliver the messages that have been sitting undelivered for years. Tell them who you really are.
- Release suppressed emotions. This helps release trapped energy and lightens the load.
- Give yourself permission to shed swallowed tears.
- See yourself letting go the strings of a handful of balloons filled with all the hurt, fear and negative emotions of the past. Watch them soar into the air and be carried far away.

- Buy yourself a bunch of flowers in appreciation of the part inside you that has never given up on you and has been with you over the years through thick and thin. Let the flowers say 'thank you' to you.
- Write a letter to your partner (you decide whether or not you want to deliver it). In the letter ask for forgiveness and in turn forgive all the pretence, avoiding and holding back that has stopped the two of you really touching each other's hearts. Forgiveness means healing the hole in your heart caused by unforgiving thoughts.

Forgiveness means freedom from anger and 'attack thoughts'. *No-one can make you angry without your permission.*

People often blame others for the choices and decisions they have made. When you believe that a person or an event has caused your feelings, you have put that person or event in charge of you. You give away your right of free will every time you think others are making you act or feel in a certain way.

Each of us carries around inside us an image of how the world should work. We are conscious of some aspects of this image and unconscious of others. Do you have an image of what a good husband looks like? What is your expectation of a good family? What would a good day look like for you? You probably have images of all these but don't think consciously of them. We see the world not as it is but how we think it should be. This lens alters everything we see. When expectations are not met, we become upset because the world did not work out as we thought it should.

When you feel powerless you are likely to blame someone else. *Upset* is an inside job. You are never upset for the reason you think is one of the tenets of Attitudinal Healing (see below). You create danger every time you blame someone else for your upset. Remember there is a frightened person hiding beneath your blaming. If you are willing to let go of '*my way*', love will find a way. It does take courage to take responsibility for your choices, feelings and actions. It requires you to become an adult in charge of your own perceptions. I often see women who have got into the habit of 'not being' a person. For so long they have had meals at times that suit their husband and family. They have cooked what others like. When they go out for a meal they let their husband choose the restaurant and so on. Notice how often you adopt the 'I don't know, I don't care' attitude. It allows you to avoid making choices. Watch how often in one day you say 'should', 'must', 'have to' or 'ought to'. Start by changing your 'shoulds' into 'coulds' and then choose whether you will or will not. These are just small steps in themselves but they make a huge difference to your self-esteem.

Principles of Attitudinal Healing

1. The essence of our being is love.
2. Health is inner peace. Healing is letting go of fear.
3. Giving and receiving are the same.
4. We can let go of the past and the future.
5. Now is the only time there is and each instant is for giving.
6. We can learn to love ourselves and others by forgiving rather than judging.
7. We can become love finders rather than fault finders.
8. We can choose and direct ourselves to be peaceful inside regardless of what is happening outside.
9. We are students and teachers to each other.
10. We can focus on the whole of life rather than the fragments.
11. Since love is eternal, death need not be viewed as fearful.
12. We can always perceive ourselves and others as either extending love, or giving a cry for help.

It will help you to feel more powerful if you begin to own your own emotions. Look on your feelings as navigational instruments to guide you. If your feelings create a sense of peace you are coming from a place of love. If your feelings create a sense of discomfort know that you have shifted from love to fear. Holding onto anger interferes with your ability to experience inner peace. Be clear that your goal is peace of mind not changing or punishing the other person. A sure and certain recipe for distress is to see negative motives in others, or blame others for your upset. It feels a bit like scratching the scab off a wound to look at it again and again. Remember what you focus on is what you get. However there is a way through. *All that you need is a little willingness to want to see differently. Then in through the fractured fears love will find a way.*

Summary

- Forgiveness allows us to act from love, not from anger and fear.
- Giving unconditional love to our children allows us to weather the problems of adolescence and allows them to separate from us knowing they are loved and respected for who they are.
- Blaming others for our decisions and upsets leaves us feeling powerless.
- We can choose to feel peaceful despite what is happening around us.
- Willingness is all that is needed.

28

Finding meaning in your inner life

Love is the way I walk in gratitude.

A Course in Miracles

o you ever feel as if you are walking through an arid wasteland with your shoes filled with heavy, dry sand? When everything seems just too hard and you have lost the reason why you were doing it anyway. Most of us have some knowledge or forewarning about wrinkly skin, brittle bones and dry vaginas, but the emotional and spiritual dryness of the middle years often remains a hidden, unpredicted mystery. Then, one day, a hot arid wind blasts sand through our lush gardens. The meaning we attach to the ensuing chaos that naturally occurs, and how we label this part of our life story, will determine how we spend the middle years. This can be in thrashing around in fear, resentment and loneliness. Or we can be warmly connected to friends and family – and invest our energy in putting back into and giving to the community. Of course, there is not just one way to find inner peace, happiness and wholeness; there is only your way.

Delores was a very successful professional woman who had reached the pinnacle of her profession, receiving the highest accolades from colleagues locally and Australia-wide. She was a dynamic, attractive, bubbly mother of two great teenage children and was active in her children's schools and other community groups. Delores's perfect world fell apart when one afternoon her husband told her he was in love with another woman and would be leaving the family home for good the following day.

For the following six months she felt trapped in shame and self-loathing, became bitter and vengeful, and was a very unhappy woman. She said to me: 'My life was not meant to be like this.' She felt that her life was a sham and that she was a failure in every area, claiming that her professional success was because she had hung on to the coat tails of her male colleagues.

Our society does not encourage in us the desire to develop the basic skills of creating an inner life. In fact, we are living in a time when the importance of spirituality, self-awareness and emotional maturity are undervalued at best and devalued at worst. It often takes a fall in the mud or one of life's 'taps on the shoulder' before we are ready to look inside for our answers. In other words, when all the outside solutions that we have gone to in the past cease to provide us with solution or solace, we are forced, courage in hand, to turn inward for our answers and our meaning.

There was no other way for Delores to go except into the eye of the storm. I knew that by descending into the centre of her turmoil, instead of fighting it, she would eventually find inner peace. With help and encouragement from me not to judge any feeling or thought, Delores began to allow herself to feel some of her perceived worthlessness, shame and failure. The very feelings that she had been avoiding had driven her to be such a high achiever and so 'perfect' in every way possible. She had had what family and friends called the 'ideal marriage and family'. She began to trace the origins of her feelings back to her father and two brothers. Although she was obviously intelligent, it was her brothers who received the private college education and support through their university degrees. Delores, because she was a girl, went to a local private school and was encouraged to 'see some life' and get a job before she got married. Any job would do. The fact that she wanted to go on to tertiary education was discouraged, in fact ridiculed, by her father as a waste of time and money. Delores worked during the day and got her degree part-time. She made a conscious decision to do more and be better than everybody else. By doing this she would make sure that she would never have to feel inadequate or worthless again. She'd show them!

Painful as it was and through rivers of tears, Delores began to feel the process of healing at work within. Through several soul-searching weeks of stepping through guilt and self-recrimination she began to feel her loss unburden. A renewed energy started to surge up from her core. She began to look at herself with eyes of admiration for her tenacity, strength and courage – and a different sense of self began to emerge. When she was able to move through the stages of letting go the feelings she was holding onto towards her father, in other words, to forgive him in the name of her own freedom, she began to experience inner peace.

In my practice of the past 26 years I feel grateful and privileged to have worked with a great number of truly remarkable men and women. As people sit with me unfolding their stories I never cease to feel both humbled and inspired at their ability to come up with solutions once they feel comfortable and safe in a space where they won't be judged and feel trust and unconditional love. I have noticed, even in the healthiest individuals, that midlife is at the very least a time of sweeping change and a very significant developmental stage of our journey.

Our culture is filled with negative messages about ageing. Birthday cards with humorous insults about being 'over the hill' and the need for fitness trainers, weight-loss programs, face peels, tummy tucks, facelifts and collagen creams all begin to give us the message that, whatever this ageing thing is, we had better ward it off as long as possible. We somehow feel a sense of shame around ageing.

I am very thankful to Margaret for many things, not the least of which is the fact that she is 13 years my senior. This may sound strange, but I don't have many female friends or family members to show me the 'way' through midlife and ageing. My mother and grandmother were both killed in front of our family home when I was 13 years old. My mother at the time was 38 and my grandmother 64, so my life has been devoid of close family to pave the way. In fact, for some of us, there are not many good role models for middle age and beyond. Look around you at the people you know. How many have aged successfully and happily?

Anthropologists tell us that, when a critical number of people in a culture experience similar challenges, myths and rituals are born. We need myth and ritual to validate our experiences and to help us make sense of what is happening to us so that we can move through each stage of our journey, gathering the riches and seeing the enormous possibilities. However, myth and ritual take time to evolve and the midlife experience may not have existed long enough in human history for myth to be established. For the first time in human history we now have a large midlife and ageing population. *We* will become, if we are courageous, the 'myth makers'. And it will be a future generation that will create the rituals around these myths.

Because of our lack of myth and ritual we get confused, as there is no map or signpost telling us where we are, much less where we are going. In other stages of our lives we have easily recognised signposts such as birthdays, graduations, getting a good job, marriage, buying a house, parenthood. We have also had our parents, friends and teachers encouraging us and cheering us on. However, come midlife and we seem to be alone, with very few good role models or signposts. For some women, negotiating this time is made more difficult because the availability of our normal coping skills fluctuates along with our hormones. For other women the ability to get up and 'get on with it' has gone along with the estrogen. This does not mean that they will never be able to cope again. But it often does mean that the *way* in which they have coped in the past will no longer serve them in the present and certainly is inadequate for the future.

Often the dreams and expectations of what our lives were going to be have not been met. 'My life was not meant to be like this' many women have said to me, and they feel that there is little time left to realise hopes for the future. It is then that we come to the startling revelation that we have spent so much of our time 'getting somewhere' that when we arrive we don't know where we are or more importantly *who* we are. Some keep waiting to be this 'adult' who has arrived and suddenly has all the answers!

Whatever we create in the present is automatically transferred into the future. If we want a peaceful future, we need to create a peaceful present.

However, 'Life is a journey, not a destination', and to really value our journey means staying in the present. We have to give up the 'what ifs' ('What if I won Lotto – then my problems would be solved') and the 'if onlys' ('If only my husband would be less demanding and listen to my feelings'). Now is the time to start being honest with ourselves about what we want to experience and to take responsibility for our choices. Whatever we create in the present is automatically transferred into the future. If we want a peaceful future, we need to create a peaceful present.

I have heard it said that 'Life is change; we can resist it or flow with it'; but we will probably have to learn to swim as well. However, we can do more than just learn to swim; we have the challenge and the choice to move beyond our own personal stories. Looking at the big picture gives a perspective and wisdom gained from hindsight, so that we can at last give meaning to the many acts of our life's drama. From the big picture we can view this period of life with respect and validate the multiple skills and the breadth of knowledge we hold. As well, we have seen and felt change in ourselves, and thus are able to give the most practical counsel and offer the most far-seeing visions that can give our own and future generations flexibility, compassion and hope.

At this powerful stage in our development we are given access to refreshing and healing rains for our desert – rains that can soothe and make sense of confusion, heal splits in past relationships and wash away the boundaries between body and soul. They bring hope to our spirits, empower our bodies, and help us to talk about age and deal with its terrors and fears.

We can begin to balance means with meaning, power with purpose, body and matter with mind and spirit, thus giving us the potential of new ways of being, knowing and acting. We have the privilege of becoming torchbearers of a flame of wisdom so that we are ready to pass to the next generation hope to make rituals from our myths, compassion to care for our families and communities, and love to bring peace to our world.

Summary

- Facing emotional and spiritual emptiness and disappointment in how our lives have turned out can be one of the major challenges of midlife.
- Deep soul-searching is sometimes necessary to let go of negative feelings we have towards others. This and forgiveness of those who have hurt us, and ourselves, is the only way we will eventually experience inner peace.
- Myth and ritual can help us with the crises we all experience during our life journeys. It is these that need to be developed as our population ages to support us through our middle and later years.

Authors' notes

Page 13 'Professor Susan Davis ... recently made a plea ... to "Stop bombarding women with HRT" ...': Davis, S, *Australian Doctor*, c. 2000.

Page 14 'So in this sense they have not been proven to cause cancer, but will certainly make estrogen-sensitive cancers grow more rapidly': Wren, BG, *Menopause*, Oxford University Press, Oxford, 2000. He wrote 'hormones do not initiate oncogenic mutations'.

Page 19 'Victor Frankl ... wrote a book called *Man's Search for Meaning*': Frankel, Victor E, *Man's Search for Meaning*, Washington Square Press, New York, 1963.

Page 27 'This contradicts the claims of progesterone protagonists who have taken up the work of Dr John Lee ...': Lee, Dr John, *What Your Doctor May Not Tell You About Your Menopause*, Warner Books, 2004.

Page 27 'However, in a small study conducted by my colleagues and me five years ago, we were unable to reproduce his results': O'Leary, P & Smith, M, *Clinical Endocrinology*, vol. 53, no. 5, 2000, pp. 615–20.

Page 38 'We recommend the book, *Power over Panic* ...': Fox, Bronwyn, *Power over Panic*, Alpha Books, Australia, 2001.

Page 42 'Recently, a synthetic compound called tibolone has become available [which] mimics some of the effects of estrogen and testosterone, and so can relieve symptoms like hot flushes ...': Supporting research for tibolone: Landgren, MB, Helmond, FA & Engelen, S, 'Tibolone relieves climacteric symptoms in highly symptomatic women', *Maturitas*, vol. 50, 2005, pp. 222–30; and in particular, Kenemans, P & Speroff, L, 'Tibolone: Clinical recommendations and practical guidelines: a report of the International Consensus Group', *Maturitas*, vol. 51, 2005, pp. 21–8, <www.sciencedirect.com>.

Page 56 'Doris Lessing … says: "The dreaded menopause did not happen: my periods ended and that was it …"': Lessing, Doris, *Under My Skin*, HarperCollins, London, 1994.

Page 57 'About 50 percent of women have little disturbance and probably do not need to take HRT …': Morse, CA, *Menopause Transition: Progress in the Management of Menopause*, Parthenon, London, 1997.

Page 63 'Giving a young woman hormones to replace her loss of estrogen, in my opinion, does not alter her future risk of breast cancer …': See also Eden, JA et al., 'A case control study of combined continuous estrogen-progestin replacement therapy among women with a personal history of breast cancer', *Menopause*, vol. 2, 1995, pp. 67–72; and Wren, BG, *Menopause*, Oxford University Press, Oxford, 2000.

Page 68 'My gynaecological history would be appropriate for that fabled peasant woman …': Lessing, Doris, *Under My Skin*, HarperCollins, London, 1994.

Page 72 'Dr Katherina Dalton … and, more recently, Dr John Lee have written extensively about this …': Dalton, Katherina & Hilton, Wendy, *Once a Month*, Hunter House, UK, 1999–2004; natural progesterone reviewed on <www.womenshealthlondon.org.uk>; Lee, Dr John, *What Your Doctor May Not Tell You About Your Menopause*, Warner Books, New York, 2004.

Page 73 'Some gynaecologists and endocrinologists still believe that the *presence* rather than the absence of progesterone is the cause of PMS symptoms …': O'Connor, V & Kovacs, G, *Obstetrics, Gynaecology and Women's Health*, Cambridge University Press, Port Melbourne, 2003.

Page 73 'A group of 20 women were followed for 20 years, from age 35 to 55, by … Professor Jim Brown …': This was a presentation given at a menopause meeting at Prince Henry's Hospital, Melbourne. It was never published.

Page 91 'A report on the 1999 Australasian Menopause Society Congress was called "Getting the Balance Right"': 'Getting the Balance Right', *Changes*, 2000, a newsletter circulated to members of the Australasian Menopause Society.

Page 95 'Clinical evidence suggests that [tibolone] relieves menopause symptoms without causing breast soreness …': Supporting research for tibolone: Landgren,

MB, Helmond, FA & Engelen, S, 'Tibolone relieves climacteric symptoms in highly symptomatic women', *Maturitas*, vol. 50, 2005, pp. 222–30; and in particular, Kenemans, P & Speroff, L, 'Tibolone: Clinical recommendations and practical guidelines: a report of the International Consensus Group', *Maturitas*, vol. 51, 2005, pp. 21–8, <www.sciencedirect.com>.

Page 96 'Some osteoporosis experts have suggested that HRT could be given to women in their sixties and seventies and continued long term …': The idea of giving estrogens long term to older women with osteoporosis was discredited when the possible increase in stroke for older women on HRT was revealed in the WHI (Women's Health Initiative) study, but recent papers give reasons why it is still useful, for example, Canley, JA et al., Estrogen therapy and fractures in older women', *Annals Internal Medicine*, vol. 122, 1995, pp. 9–16.

Page 97 'Recent concerns about the progestogen component of HRT perhaps increasing HRT risks such as breast cancer and clotting are not convincing … Women on short-term therapy (less than five years) can be reassured that it is appropriate and safe': Hillner, BE et al., 'Postmenopausal estrogens in prevention of osteoporosis benefit virtually without risk if cardiovascular effects are considered', *American Journal of Medicine*, vol. 80, no. 6, June 1986, pp. 1115–27; see also Hillner, BE, 'Estrogen therapy for geriatric osteoporosis: just one ball in a complex juggling act', *Southern Medical Journal*, vol. 85, no. 2S, August 1992, pp. 6–10; and Hammond, C, 'Confronting ageing and disease: the role of HRT',<www.medscape.com/viewprogram?696?src=search>.

Page 97 'We do not nowadays claim that HRT prevents or alleviates coronary artery disease or stroke': The Writing Group for the PEPI Trial, 'Effects of estrogen or estrogen/progestin regimes on heart disease risk factors in postmenopausal women', *Journal of the American Medical Association* (*JAMA*), vol. 273, 1995, pp. 199–209; Halley, S et al., 'Randomized trial of estrogen plus progestin for secondary prevention of coronary heart disease in postmenopausal women: the HERS Research Group', *JAMA*, vol. 280, 1998, pp. 605–13; Pines, Amos, 'WHI and aftermath: looking beyond the figures', *Maturitas*, vol. 51, issue 1, 16 May 2005, pp. 48–50.

Page 98 'The HERS study (1998) … The WHI study (2002) …': As above; Writing Group for the Women's Health Initiative, 'Risks and benefits of estrogen and progestin in healthy postmenopausal women: principle results from the WHI Randomised Controlled Trial, *JAMA*, vol. 288, 2002, pp. 321–33.

Page 100 'The desire of women to maintain the beneficial systemic effects of hormones on the quality and longevity of their lives has exposed them to the inevitable problems of endometrial bleeding': Smith, SK, *Progress in the Management of the Menopause*, Parthenon, London, 1997.

Page 101 '… it was found that this estrogen-only stimulation over time increased the incidence of endometrial cancer sevenfold …': Marrett, LD & Meigs, JW, 'Trends in the incidence of cancer of the *corpus uteri* in Connecticut 1964–1979, *American Journal of Epidemiology*, vol. 116, 1982, pp. 57–67. This classic paper by an expert American gynaecologist caused alarm until it was found that adding progestogens cancelled the increased risk of endometrial cancer: Beresford, SA et al., 'Risk of endometrial cancer in relation to the use of estrogen combined with cyclic progestogen therapy in endometrial cancer', *Lancet*, vol. 349, 1997, pp. 458–61.

Page 108 'Modern studies measuring skin temperature and peripheral blood flow … have shown that flushes are not the same as blushes': Freedman, RR, 'Pathophysiology and treatment of menopausal hot flushes', *Seminars in Reproductive Medicine*, vol. 23, no. 2, May 2005, pp. 117–25.

Page 108 'Germaine Greer … says: "the process that causes the blood vessels in the surface of the skin to dilate is similar to the mechanism that makes some of us go hot with embarrassment and go red"': Greer, Germaine, *The Change*, Ballantine, London, 1991.

Page 109 'Recently, certain types of antidepressant medications in small doses have been shown to effectively relieve hot flushes for some women …': Loprinzi CL et al., 'Venlafaxine in the management of hot flushes in survivors of breast cancer', *Lancet*, vol. 356, 2000, pp. 2059–63.

Page 111 'Many people would agree with the psychosocial researchers who suggest that "the assumption that menopause is a universal experience at any level, biological, physiological or social, should be subjected to serious questioning"': Avis, NE et al., 'The evolution of menopause symptoms', in *Balliere's Clinical Endocrinology and Metabolism: The Menopause*, Balliere Tindall, UK, 1993, Chapter 2.

Page 112 'Some psychosocial researchers suggest that many of the symptoms which women expect to have and which have been attributed to menopause in the medical literature are "components in a stereotype of menopausal women rather then the actual experience in the majority of women"': Albery, N, 'Politics of the menopause', in Smith, SK, *Progress in the Management of the Menopause*, Parthenon, London, 1997, pp. 12–17.

Page 112 'It is true that reported symptoms vary. For example, those of Japanese women differ markedly from those reported by North American women': As above.

Page 116 'The description of the gradual dismantling of an intelligent mind, and the pain endured by her husband, is told vividly in the story of the brilliant English writer, Iris Murdoch …': Bayley, John, *Elegy for Iris*, Picador, London, 2001.

Page 116 'There is some evidence that estrogens may improve short-term memory': Robinson, D et al., 'Estrogen replacement therapy and memory in older women', *Journal of the American Geriatrics Society*, vol. 42, 1994, pp. 919–22.

Page 116 '… no increase in the incidence of major depression or mental functioning associated with natural menopause has been demonstrated': Dennerstein, L & Helmes, E, 'The menopause transition and quality of life: methodological issues', *Quality of Life Research*, vol. 9, 2000, pp. 721–31.

Page 117 'Hormone deficiency … has been shown to result in some changes in mood and learning ability, as well as in memory': Kumura, D, 'Estrogen therapy may protect against intellectual decline in postmenopausal women', *Hormonal Behaviour*, vol. 29, 1995, pp. 312–21.

Page 117 'Many studies done in the USA show that women who are on HRT are less likely to develop dementing illness …': For example: Le Blanc, ES et al., 'Hormone replacement therapy and cognition: systematic review and meta-analysis', *JAMA*, vol. 285, 2001, pp. 1489–99.

Page 117 '… scientists are saying that a long-term prospective trial is needed before doctors should put women on long-term therapy for the *sole* purpose of improving brain function': Davis, SR, American Society of Reproductive Medicine Annual Meeting, Abstract 0–199, presented 15 October 2003.

Page 119 'There is growing evidence that testosterone, the main male hormone, has protective effects on some brain functions ...': Davis, SR & Burger, HG, 'Androgens and postmenopausal women', *Journal of Clinical Endocrinology & Metabolism*, vol. 81, no. 8, August 1996, pp. 2759–63.

Page 121 'My friend, Susan Maushart, writes tellingly about this in her book, *Wifework*': Maushart, Susan, *Wifework*, Bloomsbury, London, 2001.

Page 122 'Germaine Greer ... has much to say on this subject': Greer, Germaine, *The Whole Woman*, Anchor, London, 1999.

Page 122 'One of the most delightful, if eccentric, women I have ever read about was reported in our national newspaper ...': See <http://inventors.about.com/library/inventors/blgabe.htm>.

Page 128 'Scientific studies of the effect of HRT on weight deny that HRT causes weight gain': Kritz, D & Barrett-Connor, E, 'Long-term postmenopausal hormone use: obesity and fat distribution in older women', *JAMA*, vol. 275, 1996, pp. 46–9.

Page 128 'Incidentally, it showed that the women who gained most weight during this three-year study were those *not* on HRT': The Writing Group for the PEPI Trial, 'The PEPI trial', *JAMA*, 1996, vol. 275, pp. 46–9.

Page 130 '... laughter has been shown to keep hearts healthy': Argyle, M, 'Is happiness a cause of health', *Psychological Health*, vol. 12, 1997, pp. 769–81.

Page 131 'Professor Lorraine Dennerstein ... says: "Happiness appears to be enjoyed by the majority of Australian women in the midlife years; this contradicts negative stereotypes ..."': Dennerstein, L et al., 'Mood and the menopausal transition', *Journal of Nervous Mental Disorders*, vol. 187, 1999, pp. 685–91.

Page 132 'Men suffer more frequently from substance abuse and hostility/conduct disorders at midlife, whereas women are more prone to develop anxiety disorders and depressive illness': Klose, M & Jacobi, F, 'Can gender differences in the prevalence of mental disorders be explained by socio-demographic factors', *Archives of Women's Mental Health*, vol. 7, no. 2, 2004, pp. 133–48.

Page 132 'Estrogen therapy has been shown to reduce anxiety and *mild* depression in menopausal women': Seeman, MV, 'Psychopathology in women and men: focus on female hormones', *American Journal of Psychiatry*, vol. 154, 1997, pp. 1641–7.

Page 132 '… given the recent negative reviews of HRT it is doubtful whether any woman would choose to use it to improve brain function alone …': For example, Dennerstein, L et al. (reporting on the Melbourne Women's Midlife Health Project), 'Mood and the menopausal transition', *Journal of Nervous Mental Disorders*, vol. 187, 1999, pp. 685–91.

Page 132 'The most recent study … was released online on the Internet six weeks ahead of publication': Hays, Jennifer et al., 'Effects of estrogen plus progestin on health-related quality of life', *New England Journal of Medicine*, vol. 348, 8 May 2003, pp. 1939–1954. This was accompanied by this 'perspective' on it: Grady, Deborah, 'Postmenopausal hormones: therapy for symptoms only', *New England Journal of Medicine*, vol. 348, 8 May 2003, pp. 1835–7.

Page 140 'In a *Time* cover story Robert Wright discussed the issues that cause sadness to become debilitating depression …': Wright, R, 'The evolution of despair', *Time*, 28 August 1995.

Page 143 'A study … showed that many older women "would rather be dead than experience the loss of independence …"': Sekeld, G et al., 'Quality of life related to fear of falling and hip fracture in older women', *British Medical Journal*, vol. 320, 2000, pp. 341–6.

Page 145 '… recent studies suggest that long-term HRT may have risks that outweigh the benefit for bones': Christiansen, C & Riis, BJ, 'Oestradiol and continuous norethisterone – a unique treatment for established osteoporosis in elderly women', *Journal of Clinical Endocrinology & Metabolism*, vol. 71, no. 4, October 1990, pp. 836–41.

Page 146 'The results of a study in Australia … indicate that 60 percent of women and 30 percent of men suffer from an osteoporotic fracture after the age of 60 years …': Dubbo Osteoporosis Epidemiology Study (DOES). Refer to the Consensus Statement on Osteoporosis published as a supplement to the

Medical Journal of Australia in 1997, <www.mja.com.au/public/guides/osteo/ostindex.html>.

Page 153 'The genetic risk of cancer, where women carry a specific gene, is only about 5 percent of all breast cancers': Karas, M et al., 'Cancers of the female reproductive system', in Rogerio Lobo, Jennifer Kelsey & Robert Marcus (eds), *Menopause: Biology and Pathobiology*, Academic Press, New York, 2000, pp. 360–5.

Page 153 'At least half of the breast cancers have no estrogen receptors, so it is not primarily to do with hormone stimulation ...': As above.

Page 154 '... stress, late first baby, and lack of breastfeeding – are thought to be risk factors for breast cancer': Eden, J, 'Risk factors for breast cancer', in BG Wren & LE Nachtigall, *Clinical Management of the Menopause*, McGraw-Hill, Sydney, 1996.

Page 154 'High fat in the diet was thought to be a factor, but this has not been substantiated in recent studies ...': As above.

Page 154 'Is the incidence of breast cancer increasing? Yes, because more cases are being picked up as the result of good breast cancer screening': Olsen, O & Gottzche, PC, 'Cochrane review on screening for breast cancer with mammography', *Lancet*, vol. 358, 2001, p. 1340.

Page 154 'The death rate from breast cancer is decreasing because many cancers are now picked up at an early stage': Reynolds, T, 'Declining breast cancer mortality', *Journal of National Cancer Institute*, vol. 91, 1999, pp. 750–3.

Page 154 'Women are more likely to die in their sixties and seventies from heart attack and stroke than from breast cancer ...': Horton, R, 'Screening mammography', *Lancet*, vol. 358, 2001, pp. 1284–5.

Page 154 '... tibolone is an alternative that many specialists believe can be used to relieve estrogen deficiency symptoms without stimulating the breast tissue': Marchesoni D, et al., 'Postmenopausal hormone therapy and mammographic breast density', *Maturitas*, vol. 53, issue 1, 10 January 2006, pp. 59–64.

Page 155 'It has been scientifically proven that the human papilloma virus (HPV) causes one type of cervical cancer': Minoz, N, 'Human papilloma virus and cancer: the epidemiological evidence', *Journal of Clinical Virology*, vol. 19, 2000, pp. 1–5; and Teede, HJ, 'An overall assessment of HRT', *Australian Family Physician*, vol. 31, no. 5, 2002, pp. 413–8.

Page 155 'A study … on a group of women aged 80 and over who had died of causes other than breast cancer showed that 25 percent of these women, at autopsy, had a previously undiagnosed breast cancer …': Teede, HJ, 'An overall assessment of HRT', *Australian Family Physician*, vol. 31, no. 5, 2002, pp. 413–8.

Page 155 'Certainly a woman who has had a breast cancer with positive estrogen receptors would be told not to take HRT …, even though studies done by Wren and Eden … have shown that giving HRT to such women did not increase the risk of cancer recurrence over that of a group who did not take HRT': Eden, JA et al., 'A case control study of combined continuous estrogen-progestin replacement therapy among women with a personal history of breast cancer', *Menopause*, vol. 2, 1995, pp. 67–72.

Page 162 'Dr Alessandra Graziottin, a gynaecologist … has this to say …': Graziottin, A, 'Hormones and libido', in Smith, SK, *Progress in the Management of the Menopause*, Parthenon, London, 1997.

Page 162 '… hormone therapy has an important role in preserving sexual function': As above.

Page 163 'Germaine Greer … says: "Those of us who have experienced the waning of desire as a liberation are beyond redemption"': As above.

Page 163 'Germaine Greer also says, "In sex, as in everything else, we imposed a performance ethic"': Greer, Germaine, *The Whole Woman*, Anchor, London, 1999.

Page 169 '…"with time love becomes the vehicle…"': Houston, Jean, *The Search for the Beloved: Journeys in Sacred Psychology*, JP Tarcher, Los Angeles, 1987.

Page 185 'In a study … Davis showed that administering testosterone via a patch to premenopausal women with low testosterone levels relieved many of the symptoms that had been named premenstrual syndrome …': Davis, SR,

'Androgen treatment in women', *Medical Journal of Australia*, vol. 170, 1999, pp. 545–9. Professor Davis is from the Jean Hailes Centre, Melbourne.

Page 188 'A recent study ... says that there is no correlation between androgen ... levels and sexual function in women': Davis, SR et al., 'Circulating androgen levels and self-reported sexual function in women', *JAMA*, vol. 294, 2005, pp. 91–6.

Page 225 'The following story, written by Don Gowey ... is from his book ...': Goewey, Don, *Fishing for Fallen Light*, Wakan Press, USA, 1998.

Acknowledgements

We thank all the women who gave us their stories, in particular Sonja Kitcher, a friend and client who first suggested two years ago that we write women's stories of their journey through midlife. When she said that women are not sure whether what is happening to them at this time is due to hormones or other things, the title of the book was born. Her group of friends and supporters then put together a questionnaire, which helped them to put their own stories into perspective.

A recurring theme from these women was that they did not feel heard and their questions were not answered fully, if at all. Despite a plethora of books on the market, many questions still remain unanswered.

Many thanks to friend and colleague Dr Anne Jequier, who wrote much of Chapter 9, 'Oops! I forgot to have kids', which looks at the rather difficult area of premature menopause and age-related infertility. She is an international expert in the field of andrology, the study of male hormones and infertility. She has practised for many years in the field of female infertility and in-vitro fertilisation (IVF), as well as in gynaecology and obstetrics.

Thanks also to Dr Maria Weekes, a friend and psychiatrist, who reassured us that our dual authorship is complementary rather than confusing.

We acknowledge Dr Alessandra Graziottin, Director of the Center of Gynecology and Medical Sexology, Milan, Italy, for permission to quote her work on the human libido.

We thank child psychiatrist Dr Gerald Jampolsky, who is mentor and friend to both of us. He set up the first Centre for Attitudinal Healing in Tiburon, USA, in 1975. He was inspired to do this by the example of some of his young patients who, although dying with cancer, were somehow able to come to terms with this and live in acceptance and peace. He knew that he had to change his own attitude in order to do the same. He is now known internationally for his work for peace in countries like Bosnia.

Most of all, we thank Donatus, Mark, Craig, Lahra and Meneesha.

Suggested reading

General

Fox, Bronwyn, *Power over Panic*, Alpha Books, Australia, 2001.
Frankl, Victor E, *Man's Search for Meaning*, Washington Square Press, New York, 1963.
Greer, Germaine, *The Change*, Ballantine, London, 1991.
Greer, Germaine, *The Whole Woman*, Anchor, London, 1999.
Hendrix, Harville, *Getting the Love You Want*, Owl Books, New York, 2001.
Jampolsky, Dr Gerald, *Love Is Letting Go of Fear*, Bantam, New York, 1985.
Jampolsky, Dr Gerald, *Goodbye to Guilt*, Celestial Arts, Berkeley, CA, 1988.
Maushart, Susan, *Wifework*, Bloomsbury, London, 2001.
Northrup, Dr Christiane, *The Wisdom of Menopause*, Piatkus, London, 2001.
Smith, Dr Margaret, *Midlife Assessment: A Handbook for Women*, Caring for Women Publications, Perth, 1996.

Medical

Berg, G & Hammar, M (eds), 'The Modern Management of Menopause', *Proceedings of the 7th International Congress on Menopause*. The Parthenon Publishing Group, Lancaster, UK, 1994.
Burger, HG, *Balliere's Clinical Endocrinology and Metabolism: The Menopause*, vol. 7, no. 1, 1993.
Burger, H & Boulet, M (eds), *A Portrait of the Menopause: Expert Reports on Medical and Therapeutic Strategies for the 1990s*, The Parthenon Publishing Group, Lancaster, UK, 1994.
'Progress in the Management of the Menopause', *Proceedings of the 8th International Congress on the Menopause*, Parthenon Press, Sydney, 1997.

Studd, John, *Management of the Menopause*, 3rd edn, Taylor & Francis, London, 2003.

Wren, BG & Nachtigall, LE, *Clinical Management of the Menopause*, 2nd edn, McGraw-Hill, Sydney, 1998.

Useful websites

Australasian Menopause Society
www.menopause.org.au

Breast Cancer
www.breastcancer.org

Caring for Women (Margaret Smith)
www.caringforwomen.com.au

Jean Hailes Menopause Centre
www.jeanhailes.org.au

Life Focus (Patricia Michalka)
www.lifefocus.com.au

Medscape Women's Health
www.womenshealth.medscape.com

Menopause – myths and medicine
www.abc.net.au/science/menopause

The Midlife Health Page
www.midlife-passages.com

The Midlife Health Page – female menopause
www.midlife-passages.com/menopause.htm

NAMS (North American Menopause Society)
www.menopause.org

Osteoporosis
www.osteoporosis.org.au

Phytoestrogens
www.mcl.tulane.edu/ecme/eehome/basics/phytoestrogens

Wellness Web – The Patients Network
www.seekwellness.com

Margaret's story –
why hormones are important to me

Understanding female hormones and their effects seems to have become the main goal of my life. So how did this come about?

Medicine did not teach me much about being a woman. Medicine was a masculine pursuit at the time I trained in Adelaide 50 years ago. We had only four women graduates in a class of eighty. We were not encouraged to specialise and were even denied first-year residencies. They told us to go away and have babies, that we were a waste of time and resources training because we did not have the required stamina.

Fortunately, I ignored this advice. In fact it goaded me on to succeed whatever the cost. And there was a cost – I did not have children. They could not be fitted into my busy work schedule. I regret this now when I see women working in the medical field who have both a family and a career.

In the early days we had to go overseas to do postgraduate training, as there was no college of Obstetrics and Gynaecology in Australia. That came in 1978. I trained in Edinburgh for four years and did very well in my postgraduate exams. My gynaecology teachers were all men, and the teaching was all about surgery – how to remove the offending organs that bled and gave pain.

Before the Pill came on the market in the Sixties, hormones were not easily measurable. My practice today, however, uses hormone measurement to diagnose and treat women.

I had intended to be a teaching gynaecologist at a university but my adventurous surgeon husband took me off to Papua New Guinea where, for the next seven years, I was the sole consultant obstetrician and gynaecologist for the whole Highlands region. My adventures there will be the subject of my next book.

My husband and I left New Guinea with profound regret in 1971. We came to Perth so that he could do extended training in chest surgery, but he never did settle back into Western-style life. We parted in the Eighties.

I was welcomed into a university teaching job in 1972 and for the next fifteen years taught many generations of medical students. In 1978, with the encouragement of Professor Christopher Nordin and Professor John Martin, and the help of Dr Dale Evans, I set up the first menopause clinic in Western Australia. This now bears my name.

I am now in my early seventies and still practising medical gynaecology (no babies and no surgery now, just talking and listening).

Three years ago I had a life-threatening illness with six weeks in intensive care and almost three months in hospital. I was not expected to recover, but I climbed back out of my black hole and revised this book because I believe it has a message for many, many women. The Women's Health Initiative and other studies from America had hit the headlines, and women were afraid to take HRT and their doctors were afraid to prescribe it. As this book goes to press the findings of the WHI study have been reviewed and revised. HRT given to women in their fifties for menopause symptoms is now considered safe and acceptable. Even more importantly, it is the only thing that truly treats hormone deficiency!

My male teachers taught me the *science* of medicine. I certainly acknowledge their gift to me, but I am even more grateful to my female teachers, i.e. all the women I have cared for. I want to pay tribute to the thousands of women for whom I have been privileged to care in my 50 years of practice. You taught me the *art* of medicine.

I met Patricia when she came to me, 25 years ago, asking to have her fourth child at home. Other doctors did not think it would be safe. I agreed to supervise her and all went well. In fact she did so well that I missed the delivery, but of course she had a very competent midwife and great family support. We have worked together ever since, in Attitudinal

Healing and in the education and support of women through all their changes. It has been a fruitful association, which has culminated in the dual authorship of this book.

Patricia's story –
life was holding me in the palm of its hand

Love, loss and healing are the lessons I have learned over and over in my life. I was a cherished only child too sick to walk to school because of a congenital heart condition and weak lungs. Before the age of 10, I nearly died several times. My mother's devotion taught me that the most powerful thing all people crave is to be heard and understood. And she helped me learn deep down as a child the power of my own judgement. 'Listen you two,' I yelled at my parents, 'it's my heart and my body, and I'm going to have the operation'. And so the decision to have risky open heart surgery in 1955 when I was 10 years old was finally made.

On a policeman's salary, my father paid for round-the-clock special nursing. Secure in my parents' love, it was to be years later, when I discovered Attitudinal Healing, that I recognised the truth, at the deepest level of my soul, that the essence of our being is love. 'Being seen' with love, and encouraged, gives us the feeling that we can conquer the world. It is an exhilarating feeling. We spend so much time telling ourselves and others what we and they are not. It is more important to affirm what we and they truly are.

My childhood in suburban Sydney with my beautiful mother (a former model) and my huge, energetic and sociable father was shattered the day my mother and grandmother were struck by a car and killed crossing the road to visit our Parish priest. I was 13. At their funeral I had my first experience of real forgiveness. Up the path came a woman and a young man shaking, crying and crumpled in distress. The driver and his mother had come to beg our forgiveness. My father reached out his hand to them and so unleashed a force that would heal his anger and need for vengeance. Today, I know in my heart that our ability to forgive is the cornerstone of our freedom in life.

A week after the funeral, my mother's family – aunts, uncles and cousins who had previously welcomed us into their homes almost every weekend – rejected my father and me. I did not see them again until I invited them to my wedding eight years later. Frozen with fear, trauma and a sense of abandonment, my 'life in trust' was suspended. It would take many years and many different experiences of relationship to work my way through to the point where I could forgive them and let go of the hurt. Lonely and frightened at boarding school following the death of my mother, Sister Denise became more and more my only link to the unconditional love I had previously taken for granted. Still today, not a week goes by that I don't think of her.

When I left school to go to university, my father married a woman with four children and I was alone. Sometimes I was so afraid that I couldn't go to bed; I would pull a big armchair in front of the fire and sleep all night sitting on the floor. In this way I learned to live with myself. Yet during all this time, in a strange way I felt that life was holding me in the palm of its hand.

With no ties, at 20 I migrated to Canada, trained in social work, returned to Australia, married a Canadian whom I had met in Canada and had three children. After 10 years and much anguish we divorced. My dreams of family shattered, I felt a crippling sense of failure and struggled to begin again. I married a second time and had another baby, which was accompanied by an overwhelming sense of gratitude and hope. In a few weeks my husband and I will joyously celebrate our 25th wedding anniversary with our four children, their partners and our two grandchildren. Looking back, the wounds of my childhood, the relationships I had, the men I married, the children I brought into the world, the tears and laughter, years of therapy, endings and fresh beginnings, were all exactly what I needed to grow, to heal and to be healed. I have a deep conviction that love always finds a way, and that it was all worthwhile. I truly believe that every aspect of our life, correctly perceived and compassionately embraced, is simply an expression of a sacred push for wholeness and healing. More parts of my life are interwoven throughout the pages of this book. My hope is that in the telling of the various stories with heart and humour, the reader may find, from time to time, inspiration, warmth and nourishment. Let it be a reminder that we all are loved beyond our wildest dreams.

A selection of Finch titles

Blood Ties
The stories of five positive women
Edited by Salli Trathen
This collection of the stories of five Australian
HIV-positive women reveals how each woman
approached her predicament, and the inner
qualities she drew on to persevere. The authors'
honest and courageous writing allows us to live
with them through their struggles. What
emerges is a triumph of the human spirit
over adversity.
ISBN 1876451 297

The Body Snatchers
How the media shapes women
Cyndi Tebbel
From childhood, women are told they can never
be too thin or too young. The author exposes
the rampant conditioning of women and girls
by those pushing starvation imagery, and
encourages us to challenge society's
preoccupation with an ideal body that is
unnatural and (for most) unattainable.
ISBN 1876451 076

Bouncing Back
*How to overcome setbacks, become resilient and
create a happier life*
This practical book outlines some approaches to
cope with the initial trauma of loss and failure –
and to find ways to recover. Brian Babington's
approaches will help people who have
experienced severe loss – such as a death in the
family – or other traumatic events, such as the
breakdown of a relationship or the loss of a job.
ISBN 1876451 564

A Carer's Guide
*Helping you care for someone with Alzheimer's or
other dementias*
Rosette Teitel & Sharon Wall
This is a practical guide for those who find
themselves caring for a loved one at home
without training or support. Contact details for

many relevant organisations are included.
Rosette Teitel tells the story of caring for her
husband with vascular dementia in the hope
that what she learnt can help others.
ISBN 1876451 270

Catfight
Why women compete with each other
Leora Tanenbaum explores the roots of
destructive competitiveness among women.
From diets to dating, from the boardroom to
the delivery room, she describes how women
compare their looks, bodies, men, career
achievements and competence as mothers.
ISBN 1876451 491

Coping Well
Positive ways to deal with life-challenging disease
Rubin Battino
A practical and sensitive guide for those living
with a life-challenging disease and for those
caring for them, this book details many effective
coping strategies. At its heart is a holistic
approach to healing, integrating psychological,
spiritual and emotional dimensions.
ISBN 1876451 432

Emotional Fitness
Facing yourself, facing the world
Cynthia Morton outlines her innovative
program of 30 'emotional workouts', which
helps individuals learn how to overcome difficult
issues in their lives, care for themselves and
ultimately reach self-acceptance. They are
tailored for different stages along the path to
emotional recovery and have been successfully
used in sessions with individuals and groups.
ISBN 1876451 580

The Happiness Handbook
Strategies for a happy life
Dr Timothy Sharp
'Happiness is no more than a few simple
disciplines practised every day; while misery is

simply a few errors in judgement repeated every day.' So says Dr Sharp, founder of the Happiness Institute in Australia and author of this innovative and inspiring book.
ISBN 1876451 645

Into Adulthood
A parent's guide to life with an 18 to 25-year-old student
Dr Jean Edwards and Jenny English's *Into Adulthood* helps parents understand and deal with the stages that their children go through after finishing school and moving into post-secondary study. The authors, counsellors at two Melbourne universities, work daily with problems faced by students and know well the stresses associated with the transition from adolescence to adulthood.
ISBN 1876451 637

Journeys in Healing
How others have triumphed over disease and disability
Dr Shaun Matthews takes us into the lives of eight people who have suffered life-altering illness or disability. Their stories present empowering messages for all sufferers of disease and disability, and demonstrate the interconnectedness between physical, mental, emotional and spiritual health.
ISBN 1876451 424

Manhood
An action plan for changing men's lives (3rd edition)
Steve Biddulph tackles the key areas of a man's life – parenting, love and sexuality, finding meaning in work, and making real friends. He presents new pathways to healing the past and forming true partnerships with women, as well as honouring our own inner needs.
ISBN 1876451 203

Men After Separation
Surviving and growing when your relationship ends
Ian Macdonald
'Men often react disastrously to a marriage ending. This book gives a frank and direct approach to men's practical concerns, emotional

needs, sexuality, and the importance of clear and rational thinking. Highly recommended.'
Steve Biddulph
ISBN 1876451 610

Older Men's Business
Valuing relationships, living with change
Jack Zinn
In this important book, men aged 55 and over talk about adjusting to major life changes, their personal relationships and the challenges they face.
ISBN 1876451 335

On Their Own
Boys growing up underfathered
Rex McCann
For a young man, growing up without an involved father in his life can leave a powerful sense of loss. *On Their Own* considers the needs of young men as they mature, the passage from boyhood to manhood, and the roles of fathers and mothers.
ISBN 1876451 084

Online and Personal
The reality of Internet relationships
With the boom in Internet dating services and chat rooms, the authors, Jo Lamble and Sue Morris, offer guidelines for Net users to protect themselves, their relationships and their children from the hazards that exist online.
ISBN 1876451 173

Parenting after Separation
Making the most of family changes
Jill Burrett
So much parenting now takes place from two households, following separation. This book offers positive approaches to caring for children and dealing with your new and complex roles.
ISBN 1876451 378

Sex-life Solutions
How to solve everyday sexual problems
Respected sex therapist Dr Janet Hall offers clear and practical step-by-step directions for solving all types of sexual difficulties. The book includes sections for men, women and couples, as well as

one on anxieties based on mixed messages and misunderstandings about sex.
ISBN 1876451 408

Side by Side
How to think differently about your relationship
Jo Lamble and Sue Morris provide helpful strategies to overcome the pressures that lead to break-ups, as well as valuable advice on communication, problem solving and understanding the stages in new and established relationships. A marvellous book for young people.
ISBN 1876451 092

Stepfamily Life
Why it is different – and how to make it work
In Margaret Newman's experience, stepfamily life *is* different, and therefore different solutions are needed to get it 'on track' – and, more importantly, to help it survive. Margaret considers a wide range of stepfamily scenarios, and gives practical suggestions about what to do in each case to overcome any difficulties.
ISBN 1876451 521

A Strong Marriage
Staying connected in a world that pulls us apart
Dr William Doherty believes that today's divorce epidemic is the result of overwhelming and conflicting demands on our time, rampant consumerism, and the often skewed emphasis we place on personal fulfilment. This book shows how to restore a marriage worth saving – even when it seems too late.
ISBN 1876451 459

Take Control of Your Life
The five-step plan to health and happiness (2nd edition)
Dr Gail Ratcliffe
This book is a blueprint for recognising what is wrong with your life, minimising your stress, and maximising the opportunities to reach your goals. The author, a clinical psychologist, has developed her five-step method of life-planning and stress management with clients for over 13 years.
ISBN 1876451 513

Twelve Principles
Living with integrity in the twenty-first century
For a world seeking moral leadership, Tasmanian environmentalist Martin Hawes proposes ways by which we can live responsibly, reappraise our values, and develop a global consciousness. Includes profiles of inspirational people from around the world.
ISBN 1876451 483

Understanding the Woman in Your Life
A man's guide to a happy relationship
Steve Vinay Gunther
This entertaining, no-nonsense guide is full of relationship-saving advice, delivered with warmth as well as the occasional wake-up punch.
ISBN 1876451 67X

When Our Children Come Out
How to support gay, lesbian, bisexual and transgendered young people
For young people struggling with issues around their sexuality, 'coming out' to their families, schools and communities can be traumatic. Dr Maria Pallotta-Chiarolli has compiled a valuable guide for all those whose lives are affected by a young person coming out – parents of young people, high-school teachers and community leaders – as well as strategies for dealing with homophobia in any environment.
ISBN 1876451 440

Women Can't Hear What Men Don't Say
Destroying myths, creating love
Dr Warren Farrell provides a remarkable communication program to assist couples in understanding and loving each other more fully.
ISBN 1876451 319

For further information on our titles, visit our website: www.finch.com.au

Index

INDEX | 277

effect on whole woman 142–43
five cardinal symptoms 26–27
hormone levels 10–11
individual assessment 13
male/female hormone loss 189
management of 2–4, 14
natural transition 60
negative effects of 57
negative media exposure 56
not discussed 211
old definition of 120
onset of 3
positive effects of 57–60
premature 29, 62
significance of 3
surgically induced 28, 62–63, 65–66
varied experiences 111–12
menopause-like symptoms 27–28
menorrhagia 101, 103
menstrual cycle
chart *11*
explained 11–12
hormone balance during 73
reproductive life 70–71
menstruation
beginning of 209–10
difficult history 66
modern woman 211
not what nature intended 101
'primitive' women 211
mental breakdown, family history of 212
mental functioning 117
'mental' illness, stigmatised 76–77
middle age spread 127
midlife
changes and challenges 16–24
emotionally painful 169–70
memory loss 114–19
men reaching 52–53
new-found freedom 57–59
relationship changes 203
relationship ending 200–201
rite of passage 172–73, 176–77
migrant women
effect of childhood 136
loneliness 138–40
social isolation 40
minimal trauma fractures 145, 147
mirroring 203
mood swings 132
mood-altering drugs 76–77
motherhood

greatest gift of 203
late 212
mother's story, internalised 171
mother's verses 120–21
Murdoch, Iris 116

needed, needing to be 199–200
New Guinea
breastfeeding 150
gender roles 122
reproductive life 70
status of menopausal women 210–11
night sweats 29–30
Nordin, Professor Christopher 142–43

oral contraceptive pill
controlling flooding 104
at midlife 28–29
in perimenopause 47
period control 66–67
PMS symptoms 74
Resistant Ovary Syndrome 64–65
osteoporosis
bone density measurement 96
HRT with 1, 50, 95, 96–97
long-term management 98
loss of independence 143
prevention of 145–46
treatment of 96
see also bone density
otherness consciousness 203–4
ova *see* eggs
ovarian stimulation 66
ovarian tissue, cryopreserved 85
ovaries
induced failure of 64
intermittent failure 66–67
removal of 28, 63
ovulation
late thirties 73
process of 10
stimulation of 86–87

palpitations 37, 38
panic attacks
hormone deficiency 26
managing 38–44
symptoms 37–38
parenting, critical 51
past ways, letting go of 173–75, 182, 199, 227–29

peace
inner, steps to 172
sense of 240–41
'peak bone mass' 144
PEPI (Postmenopausal Estrogen/Progestin Interval) trial 128
perfectionist drive
critical mother 43
effect on hormonal pattern 67–69
PMDD 77
severe PMS 74
perimenopause
cycle chart *12*
explained 25–26
'going in and out' 45–48
identifying 29–31
onset of 2
reduced fertility 79–87
risk of cardiovascular disease 98
periods *see* bleeding; menstrual cycle
personality
effect on hormonal pattern 67–69
prone to PMS/PMDD 77
physical activity 142, 146
pituitary gland 10
plant estrogens 14, 109
PMDD (Premenstrual Dysphoric Disorder) 71, 75–77, 77
PMS (premenstrual syndrome) 26
explained 71–77
lifestyle changes 74–75
mood swings 132
oral contraceptive pill 74
personality and 67, 77
premenopausal change 77
Prozac 76
testosterone patch 185
treatments for 75
PMT (premenstrual tension) *see* PMS (premenstrual syndrome)
positive thoughts, daily 204–5
pregnancy
delayed 77–83, 86–87
at earlier age 86
methods of achieving 84–87
terminations 81–82
usually unplanned 80
Premarin 187
primordial follicles 85
progesterone
creams 72